FAT - LOSS BLUEPRINT
THE HIDDEN SECRETS

What The Weight Loss Industry doesn't want you to know.... – a complete guide

By Simon Brett

Library of Congress Control Number: 2016918322

Table of Contents

Foreword- Simon's Story

Hi, I wanted to introduce myself and let you know what this book is about and, more importantly, what it's <u>not</u> about. Firstly, thank you for taking your time to read this book. That means one more person gets their hands on information they actually need and a fighting chance to reach their weight loss goals.

Warning! If you are expecting me to reveal amazing new secrets about dieting, exercise and nutrition... You may well be disappointed. For one, I don't believe there are any "new" secrets, yet every day it seems a new "miracle diet" or "weight loss trick" comes out. I'm sorry to break it to you but success in losing body fat involves making some changes.... But stick with it – and it will change your life.

What I can promise is that the secrets I am about to share with you will give you the information, motivation and tools to significantly increase your understanding of body fat and how to reach your fat loss goals WAY faster. I will reveal a shocking fact that totally floored me and changed the way I approached my quest to lose weight.

You will get access to the exact same information that allowed me to lose over a stone in weight and 2 inches of belly fat – and keep it off.

If you're reading this right now, then chances are that you're a typical everyday person who wants to lose body fat as quickly and easily as possible without spending your whole life following a weight loss program.

You may have tried and failed once or many times to lose weight. You may feel desperate to lose weight. This book will help you understand why and the information I will give you is no BS, simple and actionable IMMEDIATELY!

Introduction

Sitting on a plane waiting to take off, I found myself wondering why the prospect of the upcoming flight (something I normally enjoy) was filling me with trepidation - something didn't feel right.

I was heading back home to London from Tampa Florida, and my fears were justified. Soon my eyes were streaming, nose running and I had a cough that would wake the dead! I didn't know it yet, but I had picked up a chest infection over the last few days, and this got steadily worse as the 9-hour flight wore on. So what was I doing on a flight from Tampa to London? Well let me start from the beginning.

You see, I have always been an active person and weight gain was never an issue. However, a few years on the road stuck in a car as a salesman meant a steady diet of fast food (burger joints in particular), high fat snacks from service stations and convenience stores.

And this is where my life became very complicated and changed forever. I had a full time job, one child, and my partner who was carrying our next child. A combination of stress, poor eating, lack of physical activity, an expanding waistline, chest pains and no energy meant that impending poor health was coming my way. I knew the dangers of being overweight and like so many others, I started researching the internet for a miracle weight loss system.

I LOVE herbal supplements! I take them every day – always have and I believe the right supplement truly complements and supports a healthy lifestyle – so I really wanted to find a good weight loss supplement. A few people I know had tried some of those online deals, but didn't have many good things to say about their experience. Some even had to cancel credit cards because of hidden monthly charges slapped onto their account and fake customer service numbers – give me a break!

Ignoring my family's advice, I spent countless hours on the internet researching hundreds of supplements, ingredients, companies, experts and marketing strategies to find the most effective supplement that (I hoped) would blast away all the excess fat I was piling on.

One thing quickly became clear: <u>The health industry is full of fake products and scam artists</u>. I ended up sitting where you probably are now feeling frustrated and bombarded by hyped up sales pitches from all sides promising instant health and astronomical weight loss. I didn't know who to believe.

That's when I decided enough is enough. Clearly, the weight loss industry was dominated by big players who continue to make millions off the sweat and dreams of innocent hopefuls like you and me. So who was going to make a stand and expose them for what they are doing? Who was going to put an end to the frustration and failures experienced by most people aimlessly switching from one fad diet to the next?

At this stage, I was dead set on using the information and knowledge I had gained in finding (or making) a "magic pill" (LOL!) so I booked into a conference in Tampa where weight loss experts and natural supplement suppliers would be speaking and exchanging information.

I knew I had to have a starting point or risk looking like a complete loser. I wanted to find the best ingredients to create a killer product despite having no money to spend. On top of that, when I told my partner I needed to fly to the US to meet with manufacturing companies and marketing experts to hopefully meet someone willing to work with me to make my dream come true, she wasn't thrilled. Spending all these hours trying to create my vision while she held the home together by herself was not something she looked forward to. Now, I'm even more stressed as I owe her **BIG** time.

So, off to the US I fly leaving behind my partner, daughter and a household that needs running. I knew no one there and only had my idea to offer which was going to be a hard sell. In addition, I was feeling upset and angry at the way many of them took advantage of their customers. I spoke with multiple manufacturers. I knew what to ask and look for due to my research on the reputable companies. I knew that any solution had to be all-natural. Overall, I knew how and why supplements work. I spoke to chemists and learnt about "mechanisms of action" and the safest and most effective ingredients available.

However, as you know too well, the best things come with more cost. However, if I was going to fulfill the promise I made to myself, it was going to be the best or nothing. I'm no chemist but when you speak with an ethical knowledgeable expert, you just know. Trust me, I spoke to a few "losers" and it was painful.

The formula had to be 100% natural, no preservatives, provide scientific research backing, follow GMP guidelines and be something that is safe. This wasn't easy but I was on a mission. Believe it or not, this _was_ the easy part!. The real challenge was attending the marketing seminars. Not only were they costly and time consuming, but what I learned was amazing or should I say.... appalling.

I listened to dozens of "experts" who had made millions online selling supplements. What I learned was invaluable or valuable depending on how you look at it. I learned they were all great marketers. After listening to them, I felt like I could sell sand in the desert. However, I also learned that many of them had very little depth of knowledge in what they were selling. Many used tactics that were let's just say "on the edge." Many of them made claims and promises that were impossible to believe. To top it off, they had very little commitment to their customers.

Was I staring at the dark underbelly of the weight loss industry? It was hard to tell. Too often, their customers seemed to be left to themselves after they were sold the supplements. You can imagine what that means. I was left wondering - Who was supporting them? Who was motivating them through the process? No One!

Do you see my dilemma?

I'm in the U.S. more confused than ever but my dream and idea is growing stronger by the minute. I knew I was in the right place and desperately wanted to create something special. Then a chance encounter happened....

So, before I get into that, let me tell you that I was dead set on creating a product that had well- researched ingredients which complemented each other and ......IN QUANTITIES THAT WOULD PRODUCE RESULTS! What I discovered was that so many of these so-called manufacturers had simply developed slick sales machines using smooth advertising and quoting "sexy" active ingredients with fake testimonials and mind-blowing before and after pictures to draw in the unwary. Do I need to go on?

These manufacturers only used trace quantities of the active ingredients. (Less ingredients costs less, right?) Once the unsuspecting consumer was duped into pressing the BUY button, our enterprising "supplier" would bill their card every month and hide their contact details, leading to more anger and frustration.

Now back to my chance encounter...

It's the day before I'm due to return home. I have no big deals to impress my family with, just a lot of ideas, knowledge and a great idea for a product. What will I tell my partner and how will she respond?
I'm sitting by the hotel pool observing the buzz around me. The energy is high but I'm still stuck with this quandary:

- I have the best product but what do I do with my customers?
- How do I help teach, educate, and support them as the days turn to weeks, months and then years?

Feeling depressed, I do what most anyone would do...I get an iced tea to drink and soak in some sun. There was an empty seat next to me and this guy sits down. We exchange the usual greetings and start talking. What happened next is amazing. Call it fate, divine intervention, or a miracle but... I asked this guy why he was there and he proceeds to tell me how he and his wife are interested in selling supplements online and came to listen to the experts as well.

He proceeds to tell my how he felt this was not as good as he had hoped. He knew that support and mentoring for weight loss and health was a key ingredient that was left out. He even said it felt like a big waste of time. Like myself, he appreciated the success of the experts that were here but something didn't feel right. Now he was speaking my language. I had the same thoughts and emotions. He was about to change my approach to weight loss forever. What he proceeded to tell me next floored me.......

He and his wife were both board certified doctors. They knew that losing weight is paramount to good health. They also had a strong message that they had to deliver to as many people as possible, but there had to be more to it than just creating a supplement and selling it. It had to involve personal contact, support, expertise and someone people could trust to tell them the truth.

Did I just die and go to heaven? Here was the solution to my dilemma. Not one but two experts with medical degrees that could give my customers the support, guidance, direction and leadership they would need. Meeting at the same conference, living thousands of miles apart, we each have something the other is looking for.

I have a flight to catch so it's time to make my pitch. I don't know what to expect but I have to do **something**. I just can't face going home to my partner empty handed! So I blurt out my idea and wait.

He grills me about my product, label, manufacturing company and what each ingredient is intended to do. Was I another "expert" or was I the real deal. I quickly learned what it's like to be in the presence of a real expert. I give the answers to the best of my ability. He's just looking at me, listening. Then it happens...

He tells me about a mentoring weight loss system he and his wife have developed that has helped hundreds of people lose weight. At last count, he said they have helped people lose a total of over 8 tons of weight! He mentions that he is limited by his practice and needs to reach more people. Afterwards, he tells me about the 40+ years' experience they accumulated along with anecdotal stories.

At this point, I don't know if they believe in supplements, use them or what. Then I get blown away when he tells me that the type of formula I have in mind is a supplement he not only uses himself, but had implemented with many of his weight loss clients! Could this continue to get any better?

It's now getting late and I'm going to miss my flight. We exchange contact info before going our separate ways. I'm still not sure if we were going to work together or if it was simply just a great conversation. What I did manage to get from the doctors were expert opinions on my product. They graciously agreed to research and critique my product. They gave me the expert opinion I coveted so that I could be 100% confident when I brought the product into manufacture.

Back on the flight to Gatwick, despite feeling sick as ever, I found my head spinning with what had just occurred. I realized the business I was in was not the weight loss supplement business, but the weight loss RESULTS business. That chance encounter spawned a deep friendship that resulted in many hours of communication and discussions as to what it takes to lose weight and more importantly, keep it off. Remember, I was tapping into 40+ years' experience of experience in successfully helping people lose over 8 tons of body fat! I continuously pumped them for as much information as possible. This book, and why I wrote it – was the result of that chance meeting.

As a result my outlook on weight loss was changed forever and instilled a deep-seated desire to show people who have been failed by the weight loss industry and desperately need inspiration, how I succeeded and how they can too. I want to show you if you have experienced the frustration so many have experienced, there is a way to reach your goals.

- Want to fit into that bikini? You can do it!

- Need to be able to walk for more than a few yards without feeling out of breath? We show you how you can do it!
- Want to impress your husband with a sexy, toned new look? Yes, it is possible and yes you can do it!

LET'S GET STARTED ON YOUR WEIGHT LOSS JOURNEY!

Section 1: The Mind

MOTIVATION

$$BMI = \frac{MASS\ (KG)}{(HEIGHT\ (M))^2}$$

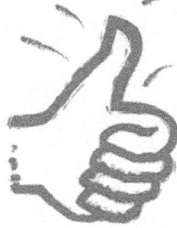

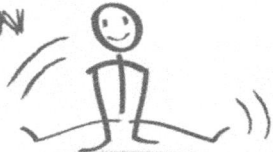

TO GO IN FOR SPORTS

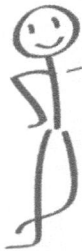

HEALTHY DiET &

KG KG

WEIGHT CONTROL

WEIGHT LOSS

DiETARY CHANGE

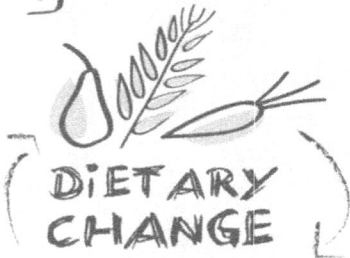

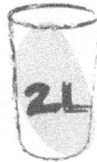

DRINKING LOTS OF WATER

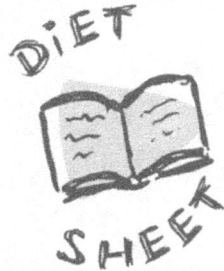

2L

DiET SHEET

Chapter 1:

Motivation, It Is What's for Dinner

As a kid, do you remember coming home after long, boring day at school to ask your mother, "What's for dinner?" Well the main course for your weight loss journey is motivation. Where your motivation lies, your health lies.

Based on that fact, this section is centered on "The Mind" and motivation is an important factor. Whenever you make up your mind to perform any type of action, there is a certain type of motivation behind it. For instance, if you're motivated to become a lawyer, you go to law school. If you're motivated to become an actor/actress, you take acting lessons and so on. So in order to become a healthier person, your motivation simply should be to *consistently* exercise and eat a nutritious, well-balanced diet, right? Correct, but it is not that simple.

You see, in terms of motivation, there are two types of people in the world:

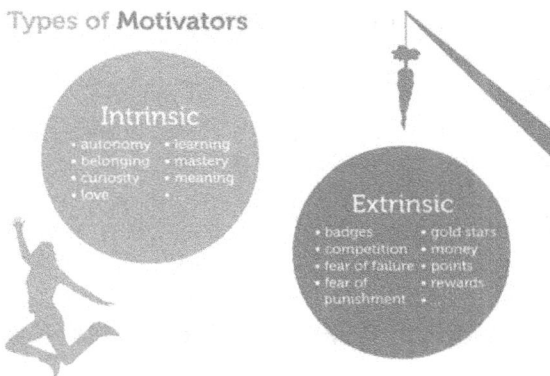

Types of **Motivators**

Intrinsic
- autonomy   - learning
- belonging   - mastery
- curiosity   - meaning
- love

Extrinsic
- badges   - gold stars
- competition   - money
- fear of failure - points
- fear of   - rewards
  punishment

1. Intrinsically Motivated Individuals
2. Extrinsically Motivated Individuals

These two types of individuals are motivated in different facets, particularly when it comes to weight loss. One individual emphatically states "I am going to lose weight" and accomplishes his or her goal. Conversely, the other individual huffs "I guess I have to lose weight" but stops trying after a few weeks. In essence, one actually achieves their New Year resolution of getting healthier while the other is face planted in a sea of glazed donuts by February. Which type of motivated individual are you? Well let's find out!

1. **Intrinsic Motivated Individual (aka Mr./Ms. Self-Motivation)**
Most people who read this book will probably fall into the extrinsic motivation category. However, intrinsic motivated people sometimes need a pat on their back in this thing called life, especially if they have recently dealt with hardships that caused their health to get off track. This type of person was me back when I was a salesman striving to take care of my family. Intrinsic motivation is when someone is motivated to accomplish certain tasks or goals to better themselves. This is exactly who people in the work world typically label as the "self-motivated" or "overachievers."

There are several traits of an intrinsic motivated person. Here are a few:
- Craves freedom and independence
- Are more task-oriented
- Are confident in their abilities to achieve a goal
- Persistent and determined to finish a task
- Enjoys learning about and exploring a particular topic or interest
- Curious about the particular topic or interest
- Relishes in mastering the particular topic or interest
- Inner drive to achieve their goal

If some or all of those traits matches your persona, then you are officially a Mr./Ms. Self-Motivated Individual.

2. **Extrinsic Motivated Individual (aka Mr./Ms. Needs A Kick in The Butt)**
Most people who are dealing with weight issues fall under this motivation classification. Extrinsic motivation is when an

individual is motivated to accomplish certain goals or tasks in exchange for a reward such as money. In hindsight, most people have been brainwashed to be extrinsically motivated. How so? School! From elementary school to college, we are taught (brainwashed) to perform a task to receive a reward (e.g., good grades, pizza party, scholarships, grants, money, etc.). That's about 15-20 straight years of being mentally trained to expect a reward for every little thing you do!

There are several traits of an extrinsic motivated person. Here are a few:

- Needs compensation to be motivated to accomplish a goal
- Afraid to fail
- Avoids taking risks
- Little to no enthusiasm about performing a task
- Needs constant encouragement to keep striving towards a goal
- Avoids conflict at all cost

If some or all of those traits matches your persona, then you are officially a Mr./Ms. Needs A Kick in The Butt.

Then Again...No One Is Completely Intrinsic nor Extrinsic

So Simon, after reading all of that motivation info, you are telling me that I am really a Mr./Ms. Self-Motivated or Mr./Ms. Needs A Kick in The Butt? Technically...yes! According to some psychologists, <u>we all are extrinsic and intrinsic motivated depending on what we enjoy to do</u>. So if you are a music lover, nobody would have to twist your ear learn to play a new instrument. On the other hand, if you care less about sports, somebody would probably cringe at watching ESPN all day.... unless someone paid you a million Dollars to do it! See how that works?

When it comes to health & fitness, some people just don't care for it. Maybe you are one of those people. Well guess what...that's okay. At one point, I wasn't too fond of working out and eating properly too. Luckily for you, I wrote this book to not only ensure that you don't make the same mistakes I made, but to receive EXTRINSIC motivation to live a healthy lifestyle. So don't worry if lifting weights doesn't give you the thrills. You will learn how to elicit your healthy side in due course.

Chapter 2: Time to Redefine the Relationship Between Diet & Weight Loss

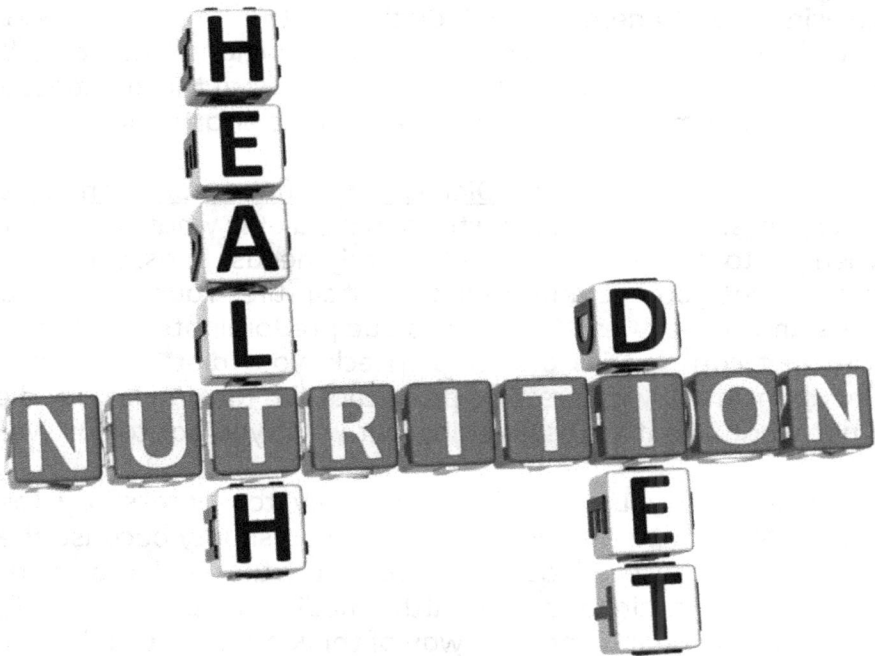

"Society has taught us that "diet" means to lose weight. When you think of diet in these terms, what comes to mind? Is it pain? Is it suffering? Is it failure? Is it something you do for a period of time and then go back to old habits? Is it something you do to reach a certain weight goal? Is it something you do to fit in?"

- Dr David Cola, "The Weight loss Manifesto"

A while back, Dr Cola *(the doctor I met at the health expo in Tampa)* and I collaborated to create an ebook called "The

Weightloss Manifesto" The book is brimming with quality information regarding weight loss and how to achieve it correctly. One chapter that really stands out is the one I pulled the above quote from, It All Starts With the "Diet." And that's the case when it comes to weight loss....it all starts with the diet.

Soooo why is dieting hard for most people?

As Dr.Cola stated, society has been taught the wrong way round about what dieting is. If you asked your family, friends, associates and enemies what dieting is, the universal answer would likely be, "What you eat to lose weight." Couldn't be further from the truth. Thinking about diet from this perspective is the reason millions of people weight loss efforts fall flat.

Let's get one thing clear: <u>Diet is not defined nor confined to weight loss.</u> From a medical standpoint, diet is what we refer to when we look at the nutrition the body needs. In essence, your diet is what you eat and drink to sustain life. Your diet can be fruits and vegetables. Your diet can be predominately red meat. Your diet can be fries and chips. Heck, your diet can even be Cinnabuns and Twizzlers! The point that I'm making is your diet is not what to eat to lose weight, but what you eat to survive.

Changing how you view diet is the key to successfully lose weight. Many men and women have failed simply because they were never educated about what diet truly is. I blame the society (the mainstream health media in particular) for brainwashing people into this way of thinking. They simply want to make a quick buck off the misery of people desperate to lose weight.

These are some of the same people who I encountered at the health expo, selling bogus weight loss supplements. Well I am definitely not a part of that "make a quick buck by selling a B.S. weight loss product" faction. This book was put together to educate and motivate you to FINALLY achieve weight loss without spending thousands of Dollars on useless weight loss products.

On that note, I will leave this chapter with ten reasons why most eating habits fail to help produce weight loss.

1. You're too strict on what you can and cannot eat

2. You temporary eat better to lose weight
This is the classic mindset of people who view diet as weight loss and vice versa. If they don't see significant weight loss in a short period of time, they toss out their quality eating plan like last year's trash.

3. You're sick of eating better
Some people get results by eating better but eventually grow tired of eating nothing but peas and carrots.

4. You have an all-or-nothing mentality
Are you the type to chuck your eating plan like a scorching baseball after eating a slice pizza? Then you have the all or nothing mentality.

5. Your metabolism is damaged
If you have a history of yo-yo dieting (losing weight then gaining it again), your metabolism is probably damaged, making weight loss a hassle long-term.

6. You use food as a coping mechanism to deal with stress

7. You turn to food when you're bored, tired, or procrastinating

8. You eat poorly because you're with friends and family
Some people feel they need to eat a bad diet because their family and friends are eating a bad diet.

9. You eat out all the time

10. You always wait till tomorrow to eat better

Chapter 3:
Revealing The Secrets of Long-Term Weight Loss

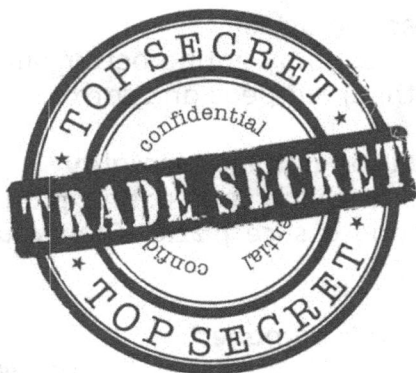

Pssst! I've got a weight loss secret for you. Actually.... I've got 50 weight loss secrets for you! The following 50 tips show the mindset and decisions of healthy, happy people who have gotten (or have always have been) in shape:

1. They focus on being healthy instead of their weight
The numero ono reason why healthy people are healthy is because they focus ONLY on being healthy.... get it? They couldn't care less about weighing a certain amount. As long as they eat well and exercise regularly, they're good.

2. They realize that getting or being healthy is a marathon, not a sprint
While weight shouldn't be a focus, being overweight or obese is not something to settle for. People who have successfully lost over 50+ pounds and keep it off takes a long-term, gradual approach to health.

3. They drink tea in the morning
Drinking tea has a wealth of health benefits including risk reduction of heart disease and boosts brain power. In addition, it's an awesome way to start your day.

4. They make their own coffee
Some of the coffees at Starbucks have more calories than a slice of deep dish pizza! That's why most healthy individuals make their own coffee minus the sugar-laden creamers.

5. They count colors, not calories
One reason some people are out of shape is they're "color blind." Filling your dish with greens, reds and yellows ensures you are making a nutritious meal that assists with weight loss.

6. They eat squash instead of pasta
If you're a pasta-loving person who desires to get in shape, try switching out pasta noodles with squash.

7. They eat wild game such as ostrich, bison, venison, and elk
Some people eat like mountain men to keep their lean figure. Wild meats like bison and elk typically contain as much protein and iron as beef or pork, but have less fat and fewer calories.

8. They drink a glass red wine per day
After a long stressful day, what's better than pouring a tasty glass of wine. Many studies have touted the health benefits of drinking red wine, including reducing depression and slowing down the aging process.

9. They choose light beer at the bar
If beer is your alcoholic beverage of choice, then make it light to minimize the caloric intake.

10. They rarely (or avoid) drink fruity sodas
It is one thing to drink sugary, Cola-Cola type sodas but it's another to drink fruity sodas. Despite the stigma that they're more healthy than regular sodas, fruity sodas tend to carry way more sugar than their cola counterparts.

11. They eat a peanut butter and jelly sandwich after a strenuous workout

Who said Pb & J sandwiches were just for kids? They are still a quality food for us adults too. In addition, this tasty snack can help you lose weight. Studies show that eating a Pb & J sandwich can help with muscle building and recovery after a strenuous workout (e.g., lifting weights).

12. They practice patience

I'm sure that you have heard the old adage, "Patience is a virtue." Well...it is! When you practice patience in life, goals seem easier to accomplish. Weight loss is no different.

13. They know organic and gluten-free doesn't always mean it's healthy

Here's a gigantic secret that most food companies don't want you to know: <u>Not everything that's gluten-free and organic is healthy.</u> Some clever companies use the so-called health words such as "organic", "gluten-free" and "fat-free" as a marketing ploy for health-conscious consumers to buy their products. Some of these products still use unhealthy substances such as high-fructose corn syrup (HFCS) as their main ingredients. So if you think that organic Oreos are a health food, then you're sadly mistaken.

14. They use herbs and spices for cooking

You need to "spice" up your life to lose weight. Cooking with herbs and spices (e.g., cinnamon, rosemary, oregano leaves, turmeric, etc.) enhances the nutritious benefits of a healthy meal.

15. They'd rather do something active on their lunch break

While everybody else is eating lunch on their lunch break, the healthy individual is taking a stroll at the nearby park.

16. They mostly do exercises they enjoy

Life is too short to do exercises that you dread. So if you feel like a hamster on a wheel when running on a treadmill, then don't do it.

17. They get 7 to 8 hours of sleep religiously

Proper sleep is like getting a physical checkup. People know it's good for them, but they don't get enough. If weight loss and better health is your goal, getting 7 to 8 hours of slumber per night is mandatory.

18. They socialize with other healthy, fit individuals

Like the old saying goes, "Birds of a feather flock together." It is easier to live a healthier lifestyle when you hang out with individuals who live a healthy lifestyle themselves.

19. They remain active outside of the gym

Going to the gym several times per week is great but the key to getting (and staying) fit is to be active outside of it.

20. They drink H2O first thing in the morning

Want to start your day off in a healthy way? Drink a cold glass of water upon waking up. Studies show that it helps cleanse your digestive system and boosts your metabolism.

21. They are in tune with their body

Healthy people know what's good and not so good for their body. They recognize when they're TRULY hungry, dehydrated, inflamed, or even getting sick. Getting in sync with your body may take time, but when you are, it's easier to stay healthy.

22. They don't live in the gym

There's more to life than bench pressing and elliptical machines. Healthy people realize that notion. They go to the gym a few times, workout for a brief period of time (30 minutes-1 hour), and leave. You don't need to spend a lifetime in the gym to lose weight. Besides, you burn the most calories outside of the gym since your resting metabolic rate (also called basal metabolism) accounts for 60 to 70 percent of your overall metabolism.

23. They get up and stretch every 30 minutes

Because you work at a desk job doesn't mean your butt has to be glued to your seat. Stretch it out! Studies show that stretching every 30 minutes to an hour helps increase flexibility, productivity, and eases stress.

24. They keep their freezer full of frozen fruits and veggies
Your freezer needs frozen fruits and vegetables in its life. The best thing about frozen fruits and veggie is that their frozen form is their highest nutritional value point. In addition, frozen foods are often cheaper and last a lot longer.

25. They avoid artificial sweeteners
So you think that Splenda is splendid? Wrong. Artificial sweeteners have been discovered to disrupt normal bodily functions and trigger a higher hunger response in the body.

26. They plan workouts in advance
If you can make plans to go to a Beyonce concert, then you can schedule a 30-minute workout at least 3 times per week. That's what busy, fit folks do.

27. They record their favorite TV shows
There is nothing wrong with recording the latest episode of The Walking Dead. Research shows that staying up late to watch TV or Netflix hinders most peoples' sleep. And when your sleep is hindered, weight gain is sure to follow.

28. They corral their emotional eating side
Look I understand. We all have our days where life is as tasty as earthworm soup (Yuck!) That's why we engage in emotional eating. Well guess what.... it's okay. Even fit individuals indulge in a bowl of ice cream with M & M pieces sprinkled on top (Yum!) to soothe their stress occasionally. Emphasis on "occasionally." They don't let a bad day transform into a bad week which morphs into a bad month that grows into a bad year (or years). Allowing food to be your coping mechanism leads to becoming overweight or obese. If stress becomes too much, please seek professional help instead.

29. They avoid cream-based soups at restaurants
Some restaurant soups are so unhealthy that you might as well order a big juicy cheeseburger with side of oily, "artery-clogging" French fries instead. Cream-based soups are

overloaded with "belly-bloating" sodium. Healthy people opt for soups that are made with clearer broths and sauces.

30. They prepare to indulge at a party or social event
Don't be that gal or guy who avoids social celebrations because the food there won't fit your macros. Fitting in an extra workout or skipping desserts during the week can allow more room to eat freely when it's party time.

31. They order alcohol on the rocks
There's a reason mixed drinks and beer taste so darn good — they're loaded with calories and sugar. That's why it is better to order a drinks on the rocks.

32. They aren't afraid to lift some heavy weights
I still can't believe there are people that weightlifting sessions consist of curling 3lb pink dumbbells. Go heavier, please. Numerous studies show that heavy weightlifting helps burn a significant amount of body fat as well as building muscle definition. Use a challenging weight that you can do no more than 8 to 12 reps per set.

33. They snack wisely
The reason a lot of people are out of shape is because they snack too much. Sure, one little bag of potato chips won't ruin your physique. But add up several bags of chips per day over the course of a week x 12 months. That's a bunch of extra calories, yet that's how some people snack. If you snack that often, start adding more fiber-rich foods (e.g., beans, vegetables, fruit, etc.) to your meals to improve satiety.

34. They indulge in desserts.... sometimes
Who doesn't desire sinking their teeth in a chocolate deluxe brownie once in every blue moon? Living a healthy lifestyle doesn't mean no desserts. As a matter of fact, an occasional dessert should be treated as a reward for living healthy. Most fit folks know and abide by this train of thought.

35. They know a weight scale doesn't dictate their health status

Your favorite health guru may be mad at me for revealing this secret but.... WHAT A WEIGHT SCALE SAYS DOESN'T MATTER. Why is that? Because most scales don't tell you exactly where you're at health and fitness wise. It doesn't tell you how much body fat or muscle mass you have. It doesn't know whether you're dropped a couple dress or pants sizes. It doesn't know whether your blood pressure is high or low. It doesn't truly know anything about your health.... except your current weight. How helpful.

36. They practice meditation, yoga and other mindfulness exercises

Question: When was the last time you turned off your smartphone and got at least 20 minutes of peace and quiet? If you're scratching your noggin, it has been too long. Life is too stressful for you not to get your mind right on a daily basis. Research shows that mindfulness exercises such as meditation and yoga helps stave off stress and anxiety.

37. They track their walking steps daily

Have you walked 10,000 steps today? That's the *minimum* recommended amount so that you aren't considered a sedentary person. Use a pedometer app on your smartphone to track your walking steps daily.

38. They know carbs aren't the devil

Whoever said carbs are the devil also thought dietary fat was bad 10 years ago and protein was dangerous 20 years ago. Listen, the media will always look to blame some food group for the obesity epidemic. At the end of the day, it's not carbs that's getting people fat; it's the people that's eating too much of it. Also, some people would rather eat donuts than sweet potatoes. Guess what? They're both carbs! Here's the purpose of carbohydrates: To give the human body the energy it needs to function properly and make it through the day. Does that sound like a dangerous food group to you? I don't think so.

39. They don't judge others' health choices

By reading this book, you decided to embark on a healthy lifestyle. Fantastic! So what do you do if your family and friends would rather eat a McDonald's apple pie than an apple? Nothing. They're living their life and you're living yours. One thing most long-term healthy individuals realize is that not everyone within their immediate circle will live a healthy lifestyle. Sure, it is painful to watch your obese relative or friend shove apple pie down they're throat but that's their decision. Just focus on your health and hope they get onboard one day.

40. They order their salad dressing or sauce on the side

One weight loss trick while eating out is to order salad dressing and sauce on the side. This helps you control how much you put on your salad to avoid adding too many calories to it.

41. They avoid the bread basket at restaurants

The garlic bread at Olive Garden is tasty is heck which is why you should avoid them while on you're weight loss journey. Most fit folks avoid the bread basket at restaurants. If nothing else, they limit themselves to no more than 2 pieces of bread.

42. They indulge in healthy fats

You thought eating fat was bad? Not if it's healthy fat. Research continues to support the weight loss benefits of consuming healthy fats like those found in olive oil, nuts, and avocado.

43. They create homemade meals more than they eat out

If you dine at restaurants more than at home, weight loss will continue to be a struggle. Over the last 40 years, the surge of people eating out at restaurants vs.at home has led to a significant decrease in nutrient density and greater health risks. By cooking at home, you control the ingredients and portion size, two vital factors when it comes to weight loss.

44. They don't always finish their plate

"Finish your food. There are starving people in Ethiopia wishing they could take your place." If you have heard a similar mantra from your mother as a child, you probably feel obligated to always clean your plate even when you're no longer hungry. Fit folks don't do that; they only focus on reaching satiety.

45. They shop around the perimeter at the grocery store
Did you know (or have you ever noticed) that the fresh fruits, meats and vegetables are around the perimeter of the grocery store? Well now you know! If you're destined to live a healthy lifestyle, staying "out of bounds" within the grocery store is where to be at.

46. They grocery shop on Wednesdays
According to a study, only 11 percent of people shop on Wednesdays. Seems like that's the day you need to go grocery shopping instead of the weekend where the grocery store looks like a warzone.

47. They push a shopping cart instead of carrying a basket
Did you know that pushing a shopping cart increases the likelihood that you choose healthier options at the grocery store? According to one study, the strain of carrying a basket made shoppers more likely to reach for quick-grab impulse items such as potato chips since their concentrated at eye level in the aisle.

48. They know to read and diagnose a nutritional label
As you know now, because a food is labelled "organic" doesn't mean it's healthy. That's why it is essential to learn how to breakdown a nutritional label to separate the healthy from the non-healthy options. Being able to do so is one of the most important skills needed to live a healthy lifestyle. Check out this FDA article: http://www.fda.gov/Food/IngredientsPackagingLabeling/LabelingNutrition/ucm274593.htm to gain clarity on how to analyze a nutritional label.

49. They avoid anything labelled "low-carb"
Healthy people aren't fooled with the "low-carb" gimmicks. Food for thought: <u>Any food that's "low" in one thing is usually high in something else.</u> That's why a number of low-carb options at restaurants are usually high in fat and/or sodium. Don't let them "low-carb" fool you.

50. They keep their snacks under 100 calories

Question: How many calories constitutes a snack? Most nutritionists and dieticians feel that a snack is anywhere between 100 to 300 calories. That's a reasonable estimate. However, if you need to stay around 1,500 calories to lose weight, two regular-sized meals (about 1400 calories combined) with three snacks, you're overeating, especially if each of those snacks are around 300 calories.

A great rule of thumb that most healthy individuals abide by is to keep snacking calories under 100 calories to decrease the possibility of overeating. Snack on fiber-rich, calorie-dense foods such as fruits, nuts and vegetables to accomplish this feat.

Oh yeah. There is one more weight loss secret that healthy, fit individuals know......

THEY BELIEVE WHOLEHEARTEDLY IN THEIR ABILITY TO LIVE HEALTHILY!

One thing in this life that I do know is belief is everything. Believing that you are capable of accomplishing a specific goal(s) is powerful. Better yet, it's life changing! With all that said, go to a nearby mirror and ask yourself, *"Do I believe in myself to lose weight?"* Don't think about it; answer with the first thing that popped in your head.

So was your immediate response....

YES I CAN!
OR
YEAH, I MEAN, I GUESS SO?

If your immediate response was the former, you get a shiny gold star! If your immediate response was the latter, then your belief system needs a tune up. Regardless of which manner you answered, while embarking on this weight loss journey, PLEASE understand that there will be pitfalls along the way that will test your belief system. That's why it is imperative that you are willing to do these 5 things to sharpen your belief like a Ginsu blade:

1. Push past your "weight" discomfort zone

Scared to go the gym in fear that people will gawk at your overweightness? Guess what...it's a 99.9% chance they won't. Overcoming your fears of what people think of your weight issue is a necessary adjustment. To be brutally honest, most people don't even care that you're trying to lose weight (*Of course, I do*), so worrying about what they think is futile.

2. Get in shape to ONLY impress yourself, not anyone else

Time and time again, people want to lose weight or get in better shape to gain someone's affection or approval. This is not a "how to get a girlfriend/boyfriend" book but realize the following thing: <u>Nobody will fully accept or respect you until you respect yourself.</u>

Men, most women actually find a man who has a chiseled physique appealing, but they find a man who has self-confidence, a good sense of humor, and intelligence even more attractive. Ladies, while most men admire a woman who takes care of her body, he also wants a woman who is caring, can cook and respects his space (*especially when football is on*). My point is that while getting a great body could potentially attract that person that interests you, you still have to develop your self-worth in order to maintain a healthy relationship.

3. Get in shape because you want to, not your doctor

The next reason ties in with the first motive except that instead of losing weight to impress someone, you're doing it because appease someone. In this case, that appeasing person is your doctor. Now most people would think that this reason is justified because people should get in shape because their doctor told them that they got pre-diabetes. And guess what? You're absolutely right except for one small nugget: <u>That person has to willingly want to make that change.</u>

Doctors around the world are always advising people to eat a well-balanced, nutritious diet, exercise throughout the week, avoid tobacco use, seldom drink alcohol, take a multivitamin, and always be happy. Yet, for some reason, many people are overweight, smoking, not exercising enough (or at all), eating poorly, excessively drinking alcohol, not taking a multivitamin, and depressed beyond belief. Why is that? Because those people aren't WILLING to change their lifestyle behavior. Even some doctors do not practice what they preach!

When you learn that you have type-2 diabetes or high-blood pressure, you need to immediately start a weight-loss program. Still, what use is a weight-loss program if you do not care to utilize it? Not even a licensed health professional such as a doctor can convince (or scare) you into living a healthy lifestyle if you do not have the will to. You have to have a strong desire to get in shape in order to be in shape.

4. Block negative junk from your mind

As you embark on this weight loss journey, understand that we live in the social media age where B.S. runs amok. With all the negative blogging, "Instagram-ing", "Facebook-ing", and tweeting that occurs on a daily basis, no wonder most people fall off the weight loss wagon. <u>I strongly recommend that you turn off your smartphone at least 30 minutes a day and get away from the madness.</u> *(Remember weight loss secret #36?)*

5. Practice 30 days of consistency to change your behavior

A wise man once told me "If you do anything for 21 days straight, it will become a habit." Add nine more days and he is absolutely right! Doing any activity for a month straight definitely sharpens your belief system towards that endeavor beyond.... belief. While some people are born with an innate self-confidence, most of us are not so lucky. It's essential that you continuously practice changing your behavior to accomplish your weight loss goal. Therefore, <u>eating better and staying active for 30 consecutive days will greatly aid your pursuit for a slimmer figure</u>. *(Note: Later in the book, a 1-month sample workout plan will be provided)*

Chapter 4: Allow Your Ego to Be Helpful, Not Lethal for Your Weight Loss Goal

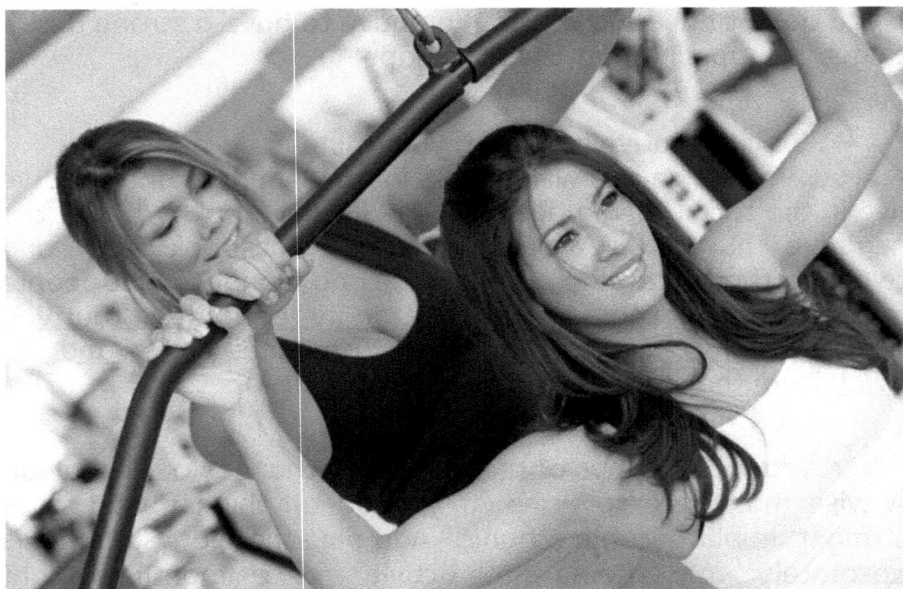

"To be ego-driven or not to be ego-driven is the question."

I had to get Shakespearean on you to discuss this last topic of "The Mind" .... The ego. The ego is a powerful motivator or a powerful deterrent; it depends on how you utilize your ego. While the definition varies from source to source, the Latin origin of 'ego' means 'I'. From this, we can infer that one's ego leads to questions such as:

- Who am I?
- What am I like?
- How do others perceive me?

So how much does the ego relate to weight loss? A lot! The ego is a double-edged sword, especially when it relates to losing weight. The same ego that motivates one to lose weight to beautify their appearance can also lead them to believing that eating a dozen Krispy Kreme donuts won't hurt.

A perfect example of how ego can manipulate a person's weight loss efforts is believing that being overweight is okay. *(A lot of women fall victim to this)* Listen, there is nothing wrong with a voluptuous woman; it's a turn-on for many men. However, if you're jeopardizing your health to be deemed "sexy" is not a good thing. *(This is similar to what I said about not trying to impress others to lose weight to improve your belief system)* So if you've got 30lb of body fat to lose, don't allow your ego – or other's stroking your ego – lead you to believe that it's okay to remain 30lb overweight.

By the way, I'm not saying being the size of toothpick is healthy...because it's not. In fact, being <u>underweight may be</u> <u>worse than being overweight</u>. Some women are naturally curvy, yet are as healthy as an ox; the pro tennis superstar, Serena Williams, is a valid example of that.

Let's go back to one of the three aforementioned questions: <u>How do others perceive me?</u> Our perception of ourselves as we relate to external forces (i.e., people, events, etc.) shapes our ego. Some people have a healthy ego; they are capable of handling a life crisis in a confident, levelheaded manner. Meanwhile, other people's egos are not healthy. These are the people who are indecisive, or not confident about how to handle a life crisis (e.g., being diagnosed with type-II diabetes). These are the people who tend to get duped by the weight loss supplement folks that I encountered in Tampa.

Essentially, these unconfident individuals allow their ego to be swayed wherever the wind blows. They allow the opinion of other's or how other's perceive them to dictate their decisions. My question to you is are you one of these unconfident people?

Here are 10 telltale signs that you lack self-confidence or have low-esteem:

1. You never stand up for yourself when dealing with conflict

Do you find yourself mostly agreeing with people simply to avoid conflict? Do you find yourself saying "Yes" to things you would rather say "Heck no!" too? Doing this is a huge red flag that your confidence is not up-to-par.

2. You always have to wear makeup before leaving the house

Some ladies get dolled up for the wrong reasons. Makeup is supposed to enhance your beauty, not cover up your low self-esteem. The same goes for guys who use expensive cars, clothes and other material items to cover up their insecurities.

3. You're unable to handle constructive criticism

Do you always find yourself feeling offended when a loved one critiques you? Lashing out at others who are ONLY giving you constructive criticism is a sign of low confidence. Sure, some people are "haters" and would rather see you sink than swim. However, ALWAYS taking criticism to heart is never a good look.

4. You're afraid to offer your opinion

Are you always afraid that your opinion(s) will alienate or infuriate others? Well... that's life. Not everybody will value nor respect your opinion. As long as you feel comfortable in your opinion, it doesn't matter what other people think of it.

5. You second guess yourself when someone gives you a compliment

A barely noticeable but apparent sign of low self-esteem is a person who always second guesses compliments that they receive. For example, if someone at work tells them they look nice today, they think well themselves, "*Why didn't they say anything yesterday? I must have looked horrible*" instead of graciously accepting their compliment.

6. You never finish what you start

You had aspirations of becoming a *(insert dream career here)* but thought it would be too hard. Giving up too soon on your dreams and goals is a sign that your confidence is lacking.

7. You compare yourself to other people

Do always find yourself "low-key" competing with other people? Comparing yourself to others is a set up for failure. Listen, because that man or woman has more money than you don't mean that they're better than you.

8. You display poor body language

When you walk, do you resemble a turtle sunk in its shell? Seriously though, a person who slouches over while walking is indirectly telling others that he/she is not happy with nor confident in themselves. You can quickly improve your body language by doing things such as keeping your head up and uncrossing your arms while conversing with someone.

9. You give excuses for your mistakes

When you mess up, do you always respond with "The reason I did this" or "I messed up because" (*type statements*?) Unconfident individuals always have to justify or rationalize every little mistake they make. If only they knew that owning their mistakes will make life much easier. We're all human so mistakes will eventually occur; just be man or woman enough to own them.

10. You overcompensate for your lack of confidence

The biggest sign of low confidence is overcompensation. Overcompensation leads people to abuse substances such as drugs, alcohol and food; thus, how most people become drug addicts, alcoholics, and.... obese. In addition, overcompensation is the reason some people express extreme attitudes such as "arrogance" and "perfectionist" to cover up their self-esteem issues.

By now, you see that it's deeper than "eat this, not that" or doing some sort of "extraordinary fat-blasting workout." Now you see that identifying and eliminating (or replacing) our own self-sabotaging beliefs and attitudes is a huge part of the weight loss process. The ego can be lethal if you allow it to be.

On the other hand, the ego can be an essential tool to engineer weight loss. How so? How can such a manipulative thing be good for your health?

5 Ways to Use Your Ego to Engineer Weight Loss

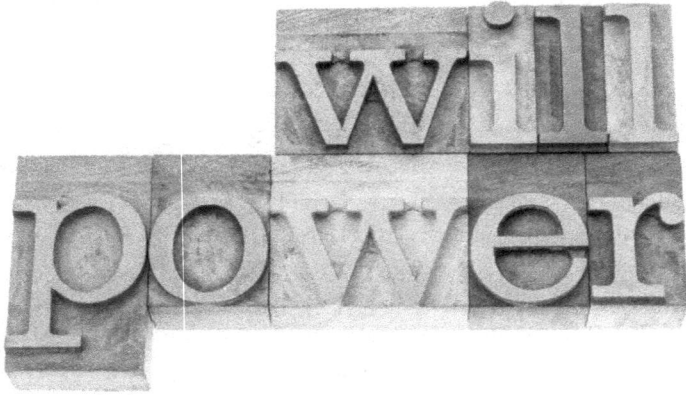

1. Allow vanity to be a motivator

Question: Is vanity a good thing or bad thing? In my opinion, vanity is not totally a bad thing...it's a wonderful thing! Vanity has spurred millions of people to go from fat to fit. The great philosopher, Aristotle, once said, *"Personal beauty is a greater recommendation than any letter of reference."* I couldn't have agreed more. By simply imagining how fantastic you will look in a 2-piece bikini or tanktop makes it easier to venture to the gym several times per week.

2. Give yourself positive affirmations (or compliments) every morning

"I am...somebody!" "I'm a beautiful person that will accomplish my goals." Telling yourself positive affirmations every morning is powerful. Let me be frank...we all have moments in life where we feel like a pile of s**t. Bad days have come and there will be more bad days ahead.

But guess what...you're still living, hence you are still very important for this lifetime. Because your weight isn't where you want to be NOW doesn't mean it won't be LATER. One of the keys to getting out of your weight rut is staying optimistic. What better way to do so than by giving yourself compliments every day?

3. Embrace your body type

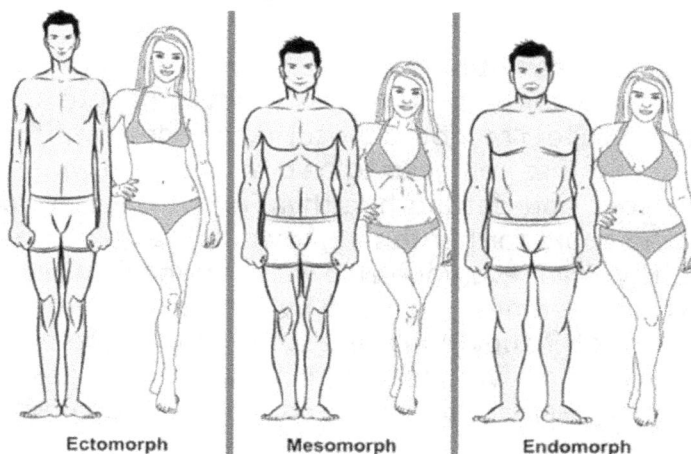

Ectomorph   Mesomorph   Endomorph

One thing that upsets me is when so-called health gurus apply a "one size fit all" to weight loss. We all are genetically different, so what may work for you doesn't mean it will work for me. Sure, most people will lose weight if they switch from drinking soda to water or from being inactive to walking daily. However, realizing your body type plays a role in weight loss is crucial. There are the three body types:

- Ectomorph aka "The naturally skinny individual"
- Mesomorph aka "The naturally athletic individual"
- Endomorph aka "The naturally heavy-set individual"

The people who have the hardest time embracing their body type while losing weight are the endomorphs because they lose pounds the slowest of the three types. If that describe you, realize that there isnt anything you can do about being naturally big or curvaceous (ladies). Remember the example I gave about Serena Williams. Get this…. she's an endomorph. If Serena didnt stay in shape, she would gain weight easily

Then again, that applies to every body type. Even if you were the mesomorph who could eat everything under the sun back in high school and remain lean, you can't do that anymore. Adulthood has a way of making everybody get their health together. So whether you will be healthy at a size 2 or 12, embrace whatever body type you are blessed with.

4. Be selfish.... sometimes

It's funny that some on the most selfish people are highly successful. While I'm not advocating to be a self-centered a**hole, sometimes you need to be a little selfish when it comes to weight loss and getting healthy. For instance, if you are a mother who cooks for her family, it would be quite daunting to cook healthy when everyone else is clamoring for fried chicken. That's why sometimes you need to cook a healthy dinner for everyone. What if they don't' eat it? Then give them money to get whatever they wish to eat. If you strongly desire to get healthy, doing "selfish" acts on occasion will keep you on track.

5. Get a pet

No, I'm not kidding. Having a Fido or Mittens can help your weight loss cause. According to a research study, pet ownership has been shown to increase self-confidence, combat loneliness, boost physical activity and instil a sense of responsibility that is truly rewarding. In addition, your pet will always be willing to boost your ego... unless you don't feed them.

From learning weight loss secrets to realizing your ego can be an asset, "The Mind" section has MENTALLY equipped you to handle your weight problem. The next section will PHYSICALLY prepare you to lose weight.

Section 2: The Body

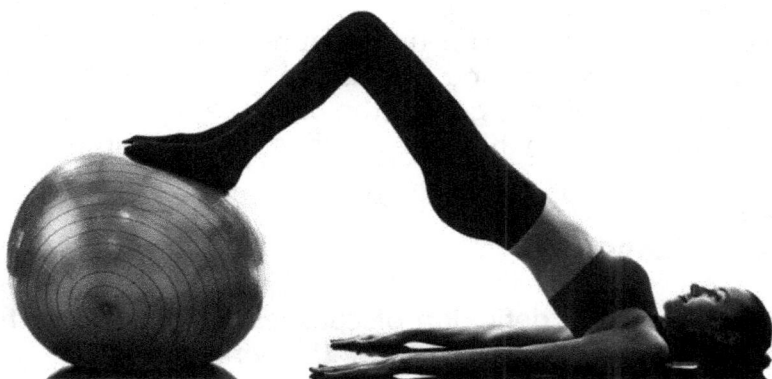

Chapter 5: The Essence of Hunger

Term: hunger
- a feeling of discomfort or weakness caused by a lack of food, coupled with the desire to eat.

Question: Do you realllly know when you are hungry? I ask this question because there are plenty of people who don't know, which leads to overeating (or undereating in some cases). One of the important aspects you need to be knowledgeable about while on your weight loss goal is the "essence of hunger." First, you must understand what are calories and how they affect you.

What Are Calories???

If you looked up the definition of calories, it reads something like *"A unit of energy needed to raise the temperature of 1 gram of water through 1 °C."* Unless you're a chemist or Albert Einstein's kinfolk, you may not grasp the meaning of that so allow me to break it down in laymen terms: <u>Calories are the foods we eat and beverages we drink.</u> Some foods have more or less calories than others, yet every food or beverage -- except water and most diet drinks -- item has them.

In addition, calories are the amount of heat produced for the body to use when food is burned or metabolized (aka the metabolism) for energy. For instance, if you eat something which contains 160 calories, it provides 160 calories of energy. If your body only requires 1800 calories of energy per day, then the fuel (food) you give it needs to be around that amount in order not to gain weight.

How do calories help our health???

To put it bluntly, if you stop receiving calories (eating), you'll eventually die. *(I am sure you already knew that but it has to be mentioned)* Without the energy that calories provide, each bodily cell will die which will lead to the heart and lungs to cease function. While obesity is a global problem, hunger (or starvation) is a huge issue in certain parts of the world too. That's why it is neither healthy nor safe to "starve yourself thin."

Getting back on the topic of food in relation to calories, there are 3 main components that most foods consist of. Below are the three main components (along with their caloric value per gram) of the foods we eat:

- 1 gram of protein = 4 calories
- 1 gram of carbohydrates = 4 calories
- 1 gram of fat = 9 calories

To get a better sense of the caloric breakdown of each component, let's examine one large egg:

- Fat: 5 grams
  5g x 9 calories = 45 calories
- Protein: 6 grams
  6g x 4 calories = 24 calories
- Carbohydrate: 0 grams
  0g x 4 calories = 0 calories

One large egg contains 69 calories total; 45 calories come from fat, 24 from protein and 0 from carbs.
How many calories do you need each day???

There is a plethora of factors that goes into what your ideal calorific consumption is on a daily basis. Some of these factors are:

- overall general health
- activity level
- gender
- weight
- age
- genetics
- height
- physical shape

As you can see, not only is it difficult to pinpoint what your basic calorie needs are, but it could fluctuate from day to day. The chart below is an illustration of rest metabolism rate (RMR) or minimum caloric requirement based on height and gender.

MEN				WOMEN		
Height (feet)	RMR Range	Mean		Height (feet)	RMR Range	Mean
5'4"	1200-1600	1400		5'1"	1120-1350	1240
5'5"	1275-1685	1480		5'2"	1135-1370	1255
5'6"	1340-1750	1550		5'3"	1155-1390	1275
5'7"	1410-1820	1610		5'4"	1195-1430	1315
5'8"	1480-1890	1680		5'5"	1235-1470	1355
5'9"	1550-1960	1750		5'6"	1270-1500	1390
5'10"	1615-2030	1815		5'7"	1310-1550	1430
5'11"	1685-2095	1885		5'8"	1350-1585	1470
6'0"	1750-2165	1950		5'9"	1370-1600	1490
6'1"	1820-2235	2020		5'10"	1410-1650	1530
6'2"	1890-2300	2100		5'11"	1450-1685	1570
6'3"	1960-2370	2160				
6'4"	2030-2440	2230				

As you can see, men generally require more calories to maintain their bodyweight vs. women. So why do the fellas get to eat more than the ladies? Muscle mass. In general, men have more muscle mass in which needs a significant amount of calories to function.... but remember that activity level plays a role too. Hence, a 6 foot, 25-year-old professional female basketball player will likely need more calories per day than a 6 foot, 25-year-old man who sits on the couch watching Cartoon Network all day.

If you're still unsure about how many calories you need per day, an easy method that some medical professionals suggest is multiplying your current bodyweight by 10 to determine the amount of calories you need to maintain the weight.

For example, if you currently weigh 180 pounds, you are consuming around 1800 calories per day. In order to lose weight, simply eat less than 1800 calories or increase your physical activity to burn more of the calories. From my experience, it is best to eat around this estimated caloric

amount and perform strenuous workouts several times week. *(Note: You'll get a sample workout plan later)*.
How do you exercise portion control or what portion size should you eat???

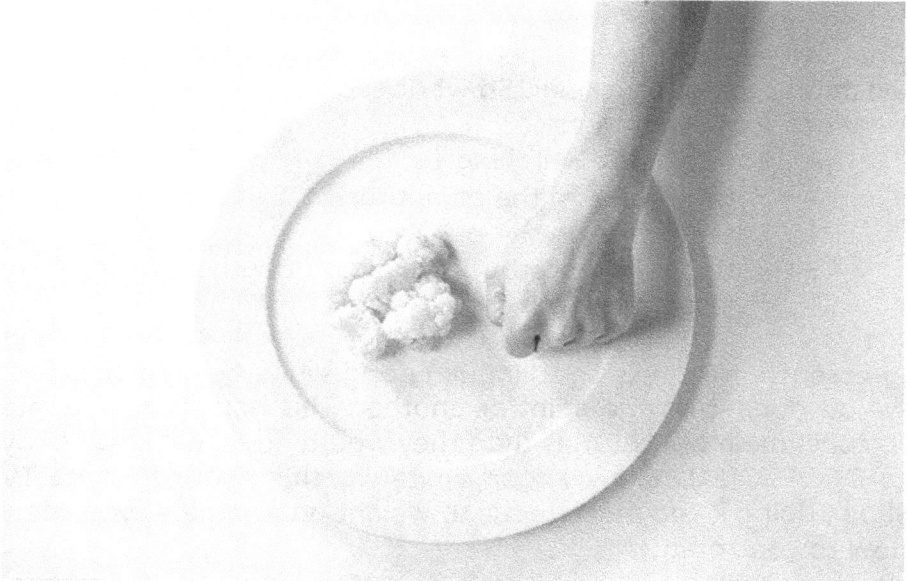

"What portion size should I eat?" "How do I measure 3 ounces of meat and vegetables?" "How in the heck do I work a triple beam balance?" Many people who desire weight loss eventually asks themselves (and health professionals) these questions.

A lot of dietician and nutritionists prescribe people these complex eating plans and be wondering why their patients are still overweight. Unless you aspire to become a professional bodybuilder, you don't need to "strategically" measure your food at all.

Besides, it's not polite to pull out a triple beam balance while out on a dinner date.

In all seriousness, you don't need measuring cups, spoons, and food scales to exercise portion control. An effective method that

I learned years ago is simply <u>measuring food portions by the size of the fist.</u> (As illustrated in the picture above) So you will have a fistful of meat, a fistful of vegetables and a fistful of potatoes on your plate. The most important thing is that you're consuming a fistful of quality, nutritious foods.

How do you eliminate mindless or wasteful eating???

One issue that keeps people overweight is mindless or wasteful eating (snacking). So what exactly is mindless eating? Here are some examples:

- Eating while watching TV
- Eating while on the computer
- Eating while on the phone
- Eating while pretty much doing anything other than focused on...eating

In essence, mindless snacking is eating while being distracted; we all done it at one point or another. This issue leads people to consume more calories than they would have. While it's okay to OCCASIONALLY enjoy food while watching your favorite TV show, doing it too much leads to weight gain...unless you knew how to control it.

Luckily for you, I have 10 scientific-based tips that helps control mindless eating:

1. Cut down on distracted eating
When it comes to consuming proper portion sizes, distracted eating is the top dilemma people face. It doesn't matter if you're watching TV, on your smartphone or listening to some music; eating while distracted can lead you to eat faster, feeling less full and mindlessly eat more. Numerous studies revealed that individuals consume more calories while distracted vs. no distractions.

2. Use smaller plates

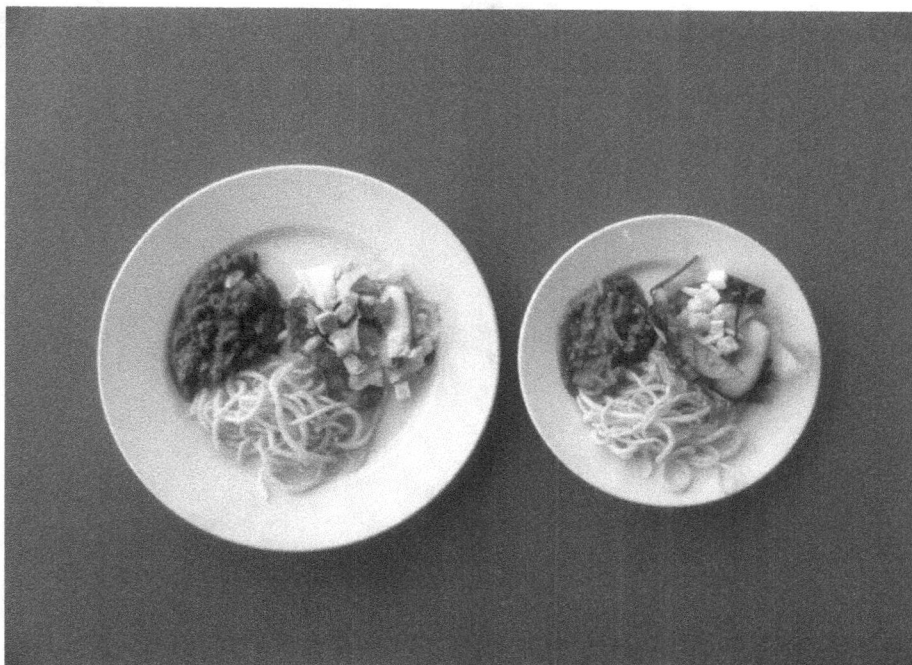

Pop quiz: In the picture above, which plate has more food? Answer: Neither, both have the same amount of food. Be honest...you thought it was the plate on the left. I did too! See the tricks our eyes can play on us? By using smaller plates, the food you place on it looks bigger.

The problem is that we are eating off bigger plates than we were decades ago, thus leading to our waistlines expanding more each year. Studies have shown that eating off bigger plates encourages us to pile on more food.

Conversely, studies have shown switching from a bigger plate to a smaller one help us consume significantly less calories. So in this case ladies, smaller is better.

3. Use tall glasses for non-water beverages

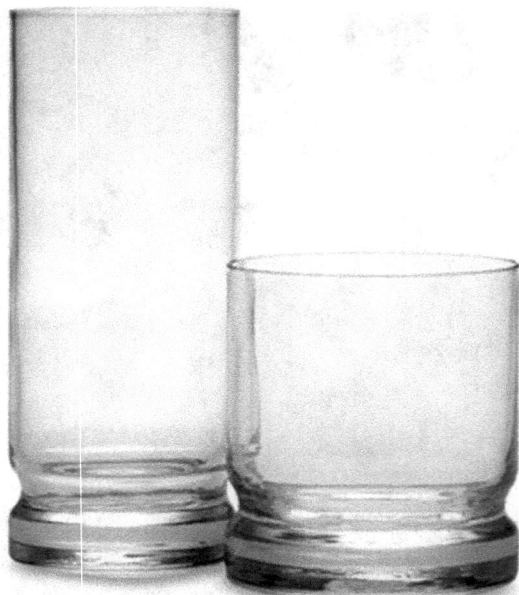

When it comes to alcohol and other non-water beverages, tall is better. Despite a tall glass and a short glass holding the same amount of liquid, studies show that taller glasses can help reduce the amount you pour by 57%. So a good rule of thumb is drink water out of short, wide glasses while using tall, thin glasses for other beverages.

4. Favor smaller packages for snack foods
Admit it! You got have a pack of M & M's at least once a week. That's fine but instead of throwing your weight loss efforts on a party size, opt for a fun size. One study showed that people who were given a one-pound bag of M & M's ate significantly more than those who were given a half-pound bag. Once again, smaller is better.

5. Leave leftovers of the food you have eaten
Did you know that leftover food could discourage you from eating more? Research shows that visual reminders of what they eaten made participants eat less vs. when their plate was cleaned. So make it a natural tendency to leave evidence of what you've eaten to stay mindful of how much you have consumed.

6. Decrease the variety of foods you eat per meal

If you need one reason to stay away from a buffet, here it is: A large variety of food encourages you to eat more. Research shows that having a wider variety of food options can lead you to eat up to 23% more. It makes sense because most people want to savor all the different flavors, thus piling their plate with as much variety as possible.

7. Keep certain foods out of sight

"Out of sight, out of mind." That phrase couldn't have been more truth, particularly when it comes to mindless eating. A study revealed that people eat more candy out of a clear bowl vs. a solid bowl. When you don't see sweets, you are less tempted by them. So if you can't help buying a large bag of fun size Snicker's, at least put it up in the back of the cupboard.

8. Eat slowly

When it comes to eating...slow down. Most people eat faster than Usain Bolt. Numerous studies show that eating pace dictates how many calories an individual consumes. Most scientists feel that taking 20-30 minutes to finish a meal allows more time for the brain to signal fullness.

9. Eat out with slow-eating people

Piggybacking off the last step, try to eat with other slow-eating people when out at restaurants. Studies show that people tend to eat more when they are with family and friends, thus the reason it is best to eat with people who normally consume food at a slow rate.

10. Eat according to your inner clock

Remember a few chapters ago when I named things that most healthy, fit individuals do? Well intuitive eating is another thing that they do. In other words, they listen to their bodies – not a certain time of day – to determine when to eat. Researchers discovered that people who relied on a certain time to eat consumed more calories vs. those who relied on internal hunger signals. Another study discovered that normal-weight individuals tend to rely less on the clock when it came to eating. Forget the outdated notion of eating breakfast, lunch, and dinner at a particular time every day; eat whenever your body tells you too.

How to determine when you are really hungry???

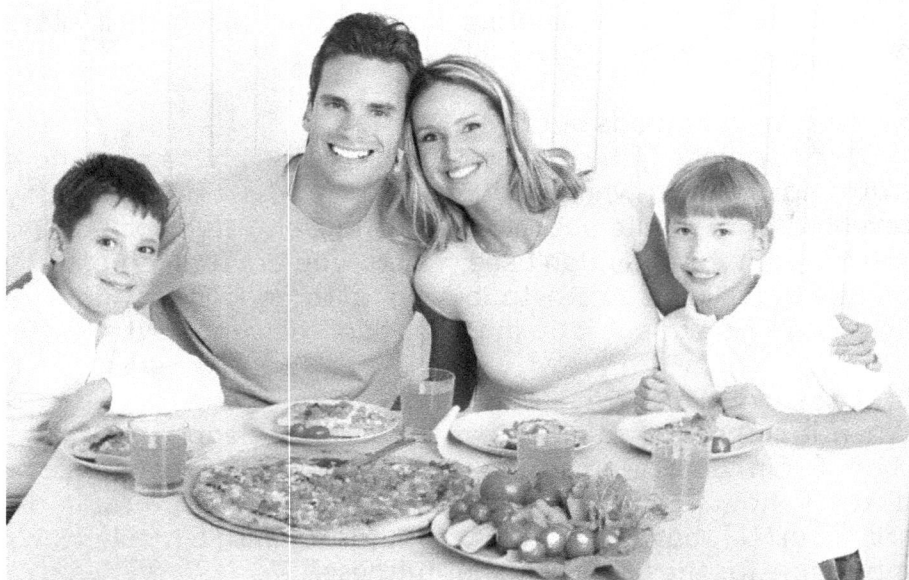

It is one thing to advise you to listen to your body to determine when you're truly hungry. However, a lot of people DON'T know when they're TRULY hungry. Here are five questions you need to ask yourself before you order (insert unhealthy food choice here):

Question 1: Am I thirsty?

Did you know that your body could trigger hunger signals when you're thirsty? Studies have shown that the human body misinterprets dehydration for hunger. While it seems that hunger and thirst should trigger two different signals, both trigger the same response within your brain. To combat this problem and ensure you're truly hungry, a water bottle needs to become your companion. The human body is made up of approximately 60% water, so staying hydrated throughout the day is compulsory. I recommend drinking at least half of your bodyweight in ounces every day. For example, if you weight 200lb, drink around 100 ounces of water per day.

Question 2: Am I craving a certain food?
A lot of us mistake hunger for craving. We all have had moments where we are watching TV and a food commercial comes on displaying our favorite dessert. Seeing that dessert makes our mouth water like a moat. Are you craving that food? Of course. Are you hungry? Probably not. If you're not sure, then take the apple test. During that moment of craving a particular food, ask yourself, *"Would I eat an apple right now?"* If the answer is no, then you're not really hungry because real hunger doesn't discriminate between foods. So please be aware of and know the difference between "crave" hunger and "real" hunger.

Question 3: Am I stressed?
In this thing called life, stress is a part of it. What most people don't know (or fail to realize) is that too much stress makes you fat. Research has shown that stress increases levels of ghrelin, a hormone that increases the appetite. In addition to an increased appetite, ghrelin causes you to crave sugary foods such as candy, chocolate, donuts and other junk food. Now do you see how stress is a "recipe" for weight gain? Remember to clear your mind for at least 20 minutes per day and do mindful activities such as meditation and yoga.

Question 4: Am I tired?
Speaking of ghrelin, levels of the hormone rises when you don't get enough sleep. In actuality, stress and tiredness goes hand in hand. Numerous studies show that when one doesn't get enough rest, they will be under a heavy dose of stress. And as alluded in question 3, stress causes people to overeat. It appears to be like this...no sleep = stress= overeating= overweight/obesity. Seems like that's the unhealthy equation many people worldwide are dealing with. Getting 7 to 8 hours of sleep per night should alleviate any sleeping issues.

Question 5: Am I bored?
One reason that's rarely discussed as a cause for weight gain is...boredom. There are some bored, lonely individuals out here who use food as a coping mechanism. *(This is the main reason*

some people have weighed 1000+ pounds!) Heck, even some of these food advertisements are using boredom to sell their products. If you're constantly overeating due to boredom or loneliness, then I strongly consider getting a pet. *(Remember the last step on how to use your ego for weight loss?).*

As you exit this chapter, I want you to become fully cognizant of your eating behavior. How in tune you are with your eating behavior determines whether you will become a weight loss success story or just another person dreaming of a slimmer figure.

Chapter 6: The Myth of Skipping Meals for Weight Loss

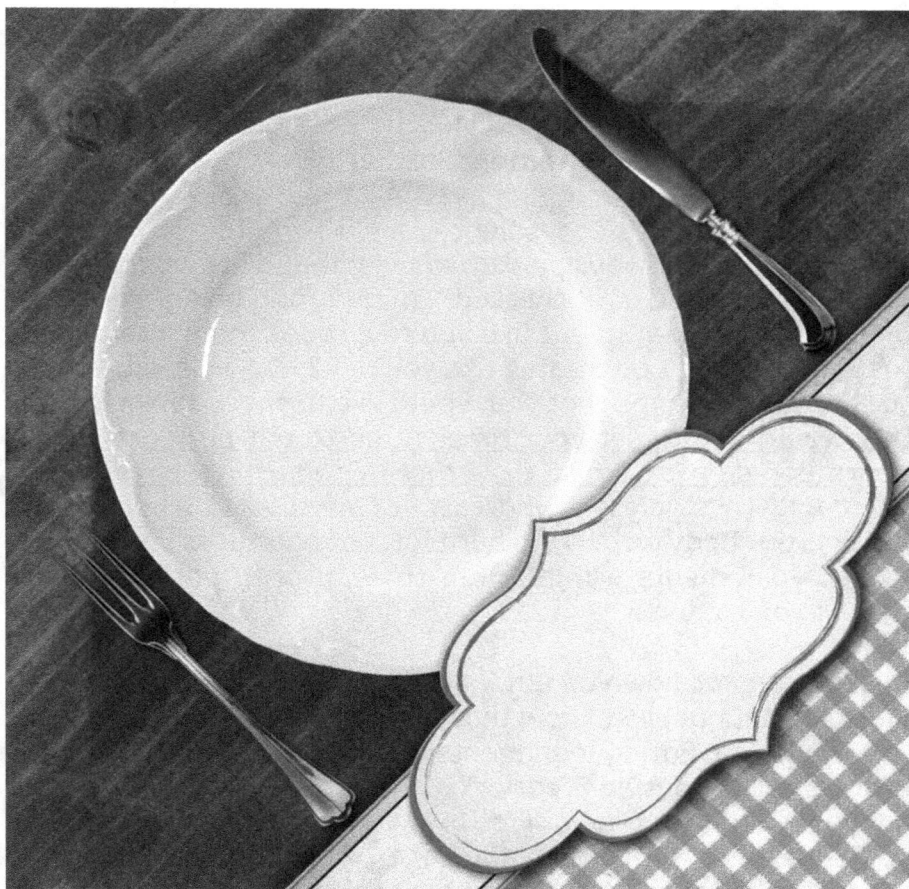

If you want to lose weight, skipping meals makes sense, right? **Wrong.** As long as the human body requires food for survival, starving yourself will never be the long-term answer to weight loss. Sure, you may lose a few pounds initially, but this presents long-term consequences to your metabolism. A study conducted on mice showed that ones who skipped meals gained stomach fat. Another study conducted on humans revealed that skipping meals during the day and eating one large meal in the evening damaged their metabolism and delayed insulin response, potentially leading to type-II diabetes if they continue to eat this way.

"Simon, what about fasting occasionally for religious or cleansing purposes?"

There is nothing wrong with fasting in this fashion. In fact, intermittent fasting (IF) is a great thing for your health when done correctly.

5 Benefits Of Doing Intermittent Fasting

1. You eat when it's convenient
One aspect that always perturbed me about diets was they told you when to eat. Last I checked, I'm a human being. Yet, these diets tell you when to eat like you're a robot. With intermittent fasting, you won't be treated like you're R2-D2. Instead, you get to set the time frame that you would like to chow down. Ideally, you would like to set your time frame to eat no more than 8 hours per day *(and fast the other 16 hours)* to be effective. According to studies, if you fast for at least 16 hours, that boosts your body's ability to burn fat. So regardless if you prefer to eat your meals within 10am to 6pm or 10pm to 6am, IF allows you to do so.

2. You can eat how you eat
Before I continue, just know that eating healthy and real food is the way to go. Eating lean meats and vegetables will make the process of losing weight easier as well as ensure you get proper nutrition. With that said, IF allows you not to feel guilty when you order that chocolate mousse or New York cheesecake at your favorite restaurant. You only get one life to live so it's okay to indulge on your favorite dessert every now and then without worrying about what some strict diet says. IF makes that a reality.

3. You don't become a slave to food anymore

One thing I noticed about people that are on diets is they become a slave to foods. Basically, they lose all their power in choosing what they will eat. Instead, they refer to a diet book of what to eat. So even if you don't want grilled chicken today, because the Atkins Diet says so, you got to eat it.

Or because the South Beach Diet told you to eat a salad right now, you go ahead and order that instead of the meatball sub that you've been craving for weeks at Subway. Guess what? You going to eventually eat that meatball sub and everything else you been craving so you might as well get it out of your system. IF allows you to stop being a slave to and start embracing the food you truly want.

4. You naturally cleanse yourself

Detoxifying our bodies is an essential aspect of health that most people ignore or is totally unaware about. Over the past few months alone, you probably compounded an enormous amount of toxins in your system, yet are unaware of it. So, how can you tell that you have too many toxins in your system? Here are 3 ways to tell if you do:

  o **You have bad breath**
If you brush your teeth (and tongue) all the time, yet people can't stand to talk to you face to face? It is because of toxins build up within the liver and colon.
  o **You are sensitive to smells**
If you have adverse reactions to smells such as cologne or cigarette smoke, then that could be because of toxins within your body. The human body becomes more sensitive to smell when the liver is unable to eliminate toxins.
  o **You are constipated**
If you find yourself having trouble doing number #2 in the bathroom on a daily basis, then that is because you have toxins in your system.

If you are full of toxins, then IF will be great for you. IF does cellular cleansing where it eliminates all the toxins in your body. That occurs because your body needs a chance to breakdown the food you consumed. It is very hard to do that if you are constantly eating. *(In which why eating 6 small meals doesn't make sense)*

5. You make life simpler
You know the key to happiness and success? No, not to strangle your in-laws that gets on your nerves during Christmas time. The key is to make life simpler. An easy way to do that is by cutting down on the decisions you make on a daily basis. With IF, you cut down the decision of when and how to eat. That's 2 decisions that are eliminated automatically! IF also helps you lose fat, maintain muscle mass, and improve your health. I'm sure those 3 things will make you happy as well.

As you just read, IF is a great method to lose weight as long as you're not skipping meals or eating one gigantic meal every day. That's why I recommended to <u>choose an 8-hour eating window that's convenient for you to eat within.</u> Once you have a set eating window, figure out how many meals you prefer to eat naturally on most days. Is it 3 meals? 5 meals? 6 meals? Figure that out because it will determine how to effectively spread calories for weight loss. Personally, I eat 3 meals on most days while I occasionally eat more or less on other days. I simply listen to my body to determine the amount of meals I consume each day.

Two Hormones That You Need to Get Familiar with: Ghrelin & Leptin

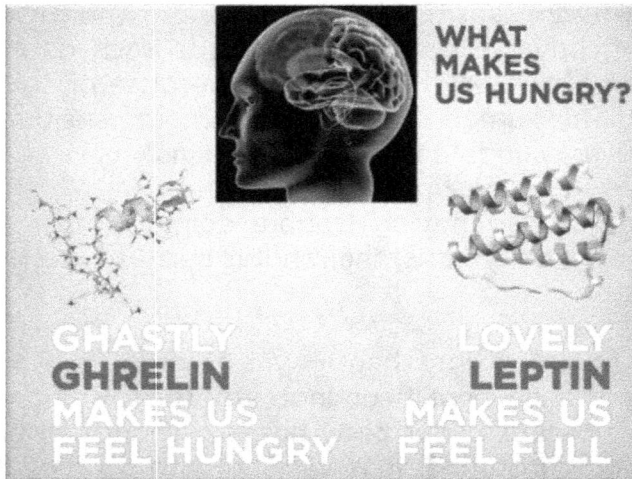

WHAT MAKES US HUNGRY?

GHASTLY
GHRELIN
MAKES US
FEEL HUNGRY

LOVELY
LEPTIN
MAKES US
FEEL FULL

As mentioned earlier in this book, **ghrelin** is the hormone that induces hunger. When the body is producing ghrelin, it sends a signal to the brain and we begin to think about eating. An intriguing note about ghrelin is that the body produces it every 30 minutes. Another intriguing fact about ghrelin is that when you skip meals, the production cycle of ghrelin increases about every 20 minutes; hence, this is what causes most people to overeat.

The other hormone of the hour is **leptin**. Leptin is a hormone in your body that regulates your appetite and how you absorb and expend calories; thus, it is responsible for signaling fullness to your brain. (So basically, leptin is Yin to ghrelin's Yang) The ironic part about leptin is it's released by stored fat. You may be thinking, *"Well that's a good thing because I have a high body fat percentage."* Not quite.

People who have a high amount of body fat tends to be leptin resistance, so they are exposed to high levels of leptin. Studies have linked high levels of leptin with a slow metabolism. In addition, leptin resistance blocks the brain's ability to receive signals that you're full. In other words, your brain is starved, while your body is obese or overweight.

"Simon, how do I overcome leptin resistance and get my appetite back on track?"

Some people have wrongfully dubbed leptin as the "obesity hormone", "fat hormone" or even the "starvation hormone." Let me tell you something: <u>Any hormone that's NATURALLY released by your body is not a bad thing</u>. The human body is designed to keep a person thriving and surviving. The body cannot help that its owner decides to give it a Big Mac with cheese and large fries on a daily basis. Leptin can be our ally or enemy depending on the lifestyle we choose.

3 Causes of Leptin Resistance

Before we discuss how to defeat leptin resistance, here are the 3 causes of it according to medical research:

1. Increases Body Inflammation

Did you know certain foods inflames or aggravates your body cells? A diet rich in sugar (particularly <u>fructose</u>), grains, and processed foods all cause increases inflammation within your body. If it the inflammation becomes chronic, not only you become leptin resistant, but other health issues such as arthritis arises.

2. Elevated Free Fatty Acids

Most people who are obese have elevated levels of free fatty acids (FFA) in their bloodstream. Not only does increased levels of FFA causes leptin resistance, but it causes insulin resistance as well, in which can lead to type-II diabetes.

3. High Leptin Levels

As mentioned earlier, high leptin levels appear to cause leptin resistance.

These three of these health issues become more prevalent in obesity. As people get fatter, these issues gets worse, leading them to become more leptin resistant over time.

How to Reverse Leptin Resistance

You may be wondering, *"Am I even leptin resistant?"* If you're overweight or obese, it's a high probability that you're suffering from some level of leptin resistance. The good news is this health problem is reversible. Here are 6 lifestyle changes that you need to implement to eventually say sayonara to leptin resistance:

4. Avoid Processed Food

Avoiding (or severely limiting) processed foods like the plague is vital to reverse leptin resistance; this also will improve gut health and reduce inflammation. (I will go more in-depth about processed foods later).

Bonus Tip: <u>Avoid any food or drink that lists High Fructose Corn Syrup as an ingredient.</u> As Dr. Cola stated in his ebook, "The problem with high fructose corn syrup is that the brain does NOT recognize this as food, meaning that when we eat this, we don't feel full."

1. Eat Soluble Fiber Foods
Including soluble fiber foods (oats, barley, beans, sweet potatoes, figs, etc.) in your diet is a good thing for improving your leptin levels.

2. Get 7 to 8 Hours of Sleep
This is the step you should be doing always; studies have linked poor sleep to leptin resistance. An increased

3. Lower Triglyceride Levels
Another aspect of being obese is having high triglyceride levels. This issue could prevent the transport of leptin from blood and into the brain. One method to lower triglyceride levels is to reduce bad carb intake (in which will automatically happen when eliminating or reducing processed foods).

4. Eat Protein
Several studies have touted the weight loss benefits of eating protein-rich foods such as chicken, beef, eggs, and nuts. There are several reasons for that, reversing leptin resistance may be one of them.

5. Exercise Consistently
"If you're not exercising, you're not surviving" should be the slogan for your weight loss journey. Research has shown that exercise may reverse leptin resistance.

As you can see, reversing leptin resistance is basically reversing your lifestyle, especially if you're obese. However, one thing you didn't see is skipping meals. This could only add to the problem of leptin resistance as well as developing insulin resistance.

Chapter 7: Workout Without Thinking About It - Tips on How to Naturally Increase Your Activity Levels

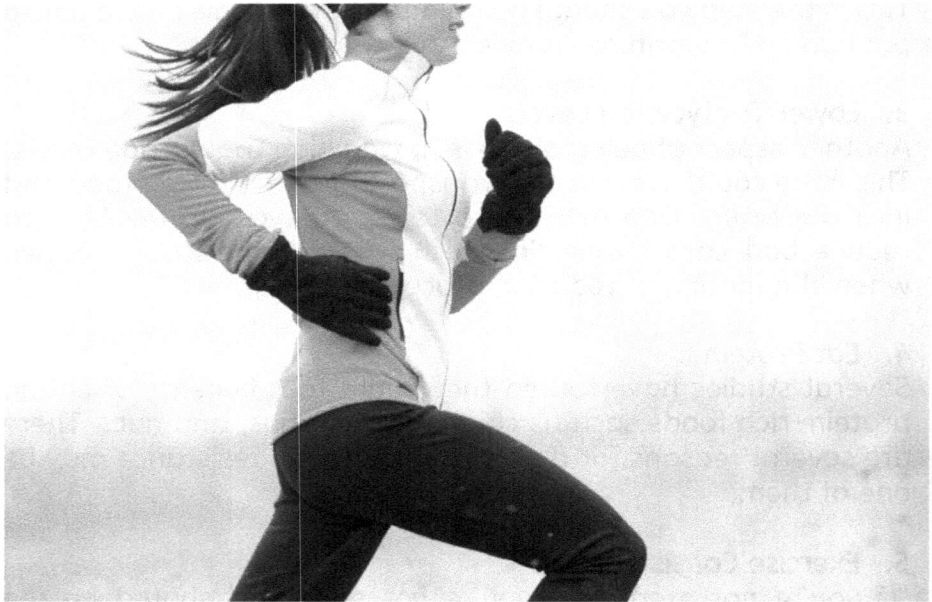

As you clearly know by now, eating habits and exercise are important to lose weight. One other piece of the weight loss puzzle that's yet to be discussed is activity levels. *"Simon, is exercise and activity level the same thing?"* Well technically, exercise is a part of activity level except it is planned.

Last time I checked, nobody unexpectedly had to perform an activity (workout) at the gym. On the other hand, there probably have been several instances where you had to do a ton of walking while running errands; this is an example of NATURALLY performing an activity.

Being active is a must to lose weight and keep it off long term. In this chapter, I will give you 20 ways that you can NATURALLY increase your activity levels. In other words, you will learn 20 ways to exercise without realizing it. Now isn't that cool? Here they are!

1. Kayaking

If you ever wanted get in shape in Mother Nature, kayaking is the answer. This activity works a multitude of upper-body muscles. Your shoulders, chest, hands, arms, abdomen, heart and back are the main muscles worked during this adventurous activity. Every row taken is equivalent to doing a single-arm dumbbell row in the gym. In addition, you can burn anywhere from 295 to 465 calories per hour (depending on your height, gender, and weight). That is many calories burnt while traveling the seas.

2. Tossing a Frisbee

It is time to get your "Frisbee tossing skills" up to par. One of the most fun activities to **boost** cardio health is tossing a Frisbee. You have run, sprint, turn, pivot, squat and jump to catch a Frisbee. With all these movements, no wonder it will burn about 200 calories per hour. Heck, I'm sweating just thinking about it! Whether you are tossing a Frisbee to your family, friends or dog, this activity will serve your heart and lungs well.

3. Take a dance class

You planning to do a dinner and a movie tonight with your spouse...again? Scrap that! Instead, you both should take a dance class. Taking a dance class not only will be good for cardio health, but a fun, romantic thing for you and your spouse to do. Here is a list of dance classes that you both should consider trying out:

- Ballet Dance
- Tap Dance
- Jazz Dance
- Hip Hop Dance
- Ballroom Dancing

- Swing Dance
- Modern Dance
- Contra Dance
- Country/Western Dance
- Belly Dance
- Flamenco Dance
- Latin Dance
- Folk Dance

4. Take a hike

When life gets too stressful, sometimes you have to take a hike. No, I don't mean leave everything behind and move to some remote island. I mean you should take a hiking trip. With so many mountains and forest trails in the world, this will be a very adventurous way to work out. Being in nature has a way of bringing focus back to people's lives. If anything, hiking will certainly bring your cardio health back in focus.

5. Rock climbing

If you're a daredevil type of fellow, then rock climbing is a fun activity to do. This activity works the heck out of your arm, back, legs.... pretty much your whole body!

6. Geocaching

If you love exploring and treasure hunting, then geocaching is right up your alley.

7. Playing hide & go seek

Who said stop playing hide & go seek after middle school? This childhood game can still be a fun activity to do, especially if you have children.

8. Kickboxing

If you ever seen one of Bruce Lee's movies, you know how well-conditioned he was. You can thank kickboxing for that! Kickboxing is an exhilarating activity that will teach you how to kick fat and kick butt! This total-body exercise works practically every upper and lower-body muscle group. In addition, your heart and lungs will be taxed after doing this activity for a few minutes.

9. Use a standing desk
If you work 40+ hours per week at an office, I strongly suggest that you invest in a standing desk. According to a study, standing caused the participants to have a significantly higher heart rate (about 10 beats per minute higher), which equates to burning around 50 calories more per hour versus sitting.

10. Have sex
Engaging in sex is not only pleasurable but aids in weight loss. You can burn up to 207 calories in 30 minutes of sexual activity. *(If ya'll last that long)*

11. Clean up your place/car/anything you own that's dirty
When's the last time you cleaned out your car or house? If you're scratching your head, it's been too long. Cleaning up is a great way to burn calories and be neat. To make the routine feel less like a chore, put on some music that make you feel alive while cleaning.

12. Practice yoga
Ohmm! Yoga is a therapeutic activity as much as it is a weight loss asset. With how stressful life can get, practicing yoga a few times per week will relax you greatly.

13. Play active video games
Who said playing video games makes people fat? There are plenty of video games that make you move and burn calories *(e.g. Dance Dance Revolution, Wii Tennis, Wii Fit, Just Dance on Xbox Kinect).*

14. Learn to play a music instrument
Which activity burns more calories: Walking around a track for an hour or playing the violin for an hour? If your answer (or guess) is the latter, you get a gold star! What many people don't realize is that our brains burn calories when it's being challenged, thus why learning to play an instrument is considered physical activity.

15. Go for a swim
Who didn't look forward to swimming as a kid? It's time to relive those days. Swimming is a fun activity to partake in as well as a superb cardio workout.

16. Join a Rec league
This activity is really beneficial if you've recently moved into a new city or town. Joining a Rec league is a great way to be naturally active while meeting new people.

17. Play at the playground
Because you're not a kid anymore doesn't mean the playground isn't useful. When on the road, it can be difficult to get to your gym, but there is always a nearby playground. A great thing about a playground is that it's the perfect place to work out when you're tired of the gym life. Besides, I know you've been dying to swing on the swing set since 1998.

18. Bike to work
If you're within a 5-mile radius of your job then, you should be consider pedaling, not driving, to work. Imagine how many additional calories you will burn per week simply by biking to work during the weekday. This will greatly aid in your weight-loss efforts. Not to mention, your legs will get super-toned from doing all that pedaling.

19. Dare yourself to do a certain amount of pushups by the end of the day
Okay, I understand pushups is a "planned" activity. However, you can make pushups a fun, spontaneous activity by daring yourself to complete a certain amount of reps every day. By doing this overtime, it will elevate your metabolism tremendously. In addition, you will build muscular tone in the upper body; especially in your chest, arms, and shoulders.

20. Take a walk
Probably the simplest way to naturally increase your activity level is to take a walk. Like pushups, the best thing about walking is it can be done anywhere. So if you travel a lot, then utilize walking, especially if it's your first time being at a certain destination. For instance, if you're in Washington D.C. for the

first time, it would be a good idea to walk around to the White House and other national monuments.

Section 3: Fat Burning Nutrition

Chapter 8: Supplement with Supplements for Proper Nutrition & Weight Loss

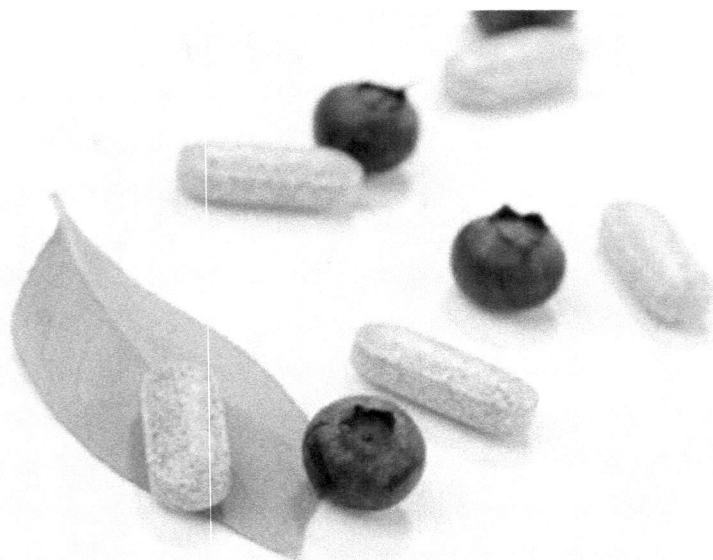

A re you getting every essential mineral and vitamin on a daily basis?

The average Western diet leaves a lot to be desired. Research finds our meals lacking in a number of essential nutrients such as calcium, potassium, magnesium, and vitamins A, C, and D. In order to maximize your weight loss efforts, dietary supplementation is necessary. The right supplement can accelerate your progress, not only in weight loss, but your overall health in general.

Now, please don't think supplements are a magic pill. With that said, look carefully at any supplier that makes any extreme weight loss claims (e.g., lose 100lb in 30 days!) as they are usually unsafe and may have serious side effects.

First thing to realize is that supplements – at least in the United States – are not considered drugs, therefore aren't regulated by the Food and Drug Agency (FDA). This absence of regulation means that the effectiveness, quality, and quantity of the ingredients have not been independently verified, which makes it important to know who is supplying the supplement.

Look out for companies that use ingredients that are very well-studied and researched.

When analyzing a manufacturer, ask yourself the following questions:
- How established are they?
- Do they specialize in supplements?
- Do they follow the GMP guidelines?
- Are they FDA compliant?

A quality supplement company will follow the Good Manufacturing Practice Guidelines to make sure that the nutrients are real, natural and exacted according to the ingredients listed.

Ingredients
When analyzing the ingredients, are you looking for high-quality authentic ingredients with little or no preservatives? Also, are you looking at the type and mix of ingredients for the synergistic effect?

"Simon, what do you mean by…. synergistic?"

The word comes from the Greek, sunergia, and is defined as 'The interaction of two or more cooperative agents or forces so that their combined effect is greater than the sum of their individual effects.' To utilize the synergistic effect, look for an approach that uses multiple ingredients that helps each other make a more potent product or a combination that supports your body's need for vitamins and minerals.

Mechanisms of Action
The mechanisms of action are how the body uses a specific ingredient to promote or support weight loss. The following are 10 mechanisms of action that you will encounter while supplement hunting:

1. Carbohydrate blocking
Overconsumption of carbohydrates is a common cause of weight gain and overeating. Carbohydrates are broken down and used by the body to produce energy. Any energy that isn't used by the body is then stored as fat. Carb blocking ingredients inhibit the action some enzymes the body used to convert the carbohydrates into energy thus causing the carbohydrates to be passed through unabsorbed.

2. Improving carbohydrate metabolism
It is essential that carbohydrates are consumed on a daily basis. The energy provided is vital for the function of the body. Ingredients in this category help the body utilize the carbohydrates more efficiently. Their desired effect is to convert the carbohydrates to energy rather than storing them as fat. Chromium as nicotinate would be an example.

3. Improving insulin control and usage
Unless you are unable to produce insulin such as the case with Type I diabetes, there are ingredients that can help regulate the amount of insulin secreted, increase the sensitivity to insulin, improve glucose tolerance and support the binding of insulin to the cells. Common ingredients that are thought to facilitate insulin usage and efficiency include chromium, magnesium, vanadyl sulfate, biotin, selenium, Gymnema sylvestre, and zinc.

4. Improving fat utilization and transportation
Fat is needed and consumed on a daily basis. Problems arise when the body is not efficient at transporting and using the fat. Instead of the fat being used as an energy source, it is simply

stored away. Storage of excess fat contributes to weight gain. Ingredients in this category are thought to speed up fat transportation, facilitate the breakdown of fat so it can be used as an energy source. Examples of ingredient's in this category include hydroxycitric acid from Garcinia cambogia, L-carnitine, methionine, and fucoxanthin.

5. Fat blockers
Ingredients in this category impair the ability of the body to absorb fat. By blocking fat absorption, the fat is eliminated in the stool. This mechanism takes place in the intestinal track; therefore, people with intestinal concerns have to be cautious. Increasing the fat content of the stool can lead to gas, cramping, bloating and oily stools. Chitosan and Cassia nomame are examples.

6. Thermogenic agents
This is the mechanism of action most people are familiar with. This involves ingredients that increase the basal metabolic rate. The rationale behind their usage is to accelerate the ability of the body to generate heat/energy. This means that calories are burned or used faster than normal.

Many people are concerned with a "slow" metabolism and look up to this mechanism to "speed" up their metabolism rate. Ingredients in this category would include caffeine, ATP, MaHuang, cayenne pepper, Garcinia cambogia, Guarana extract and green tea to name a few.

7. Appetite suppressants
This is another familiar mechanism. There has been a lot of research in this area. Studying the brain to learn the pathways associated with appetite has led to tremendous discoveries.
We know there are certain centers in the brain associated with eating. We also know there are certain chemicals produced that affect eating patterns. Influencing these centers and chemicals has led to the discovery of ingredients that can suppress or control appetite.

By choosing a safe, natural substance that affects the appetite center, hunger is decreased thus leading to the consumption of fewer calories. Ingredients in this category include Caralluma Fimbriata (Slimalum) and Hoodia gordonii.

8. Influencing neurologic and chemical balance
There is a lot of ongoing research concerning the effect of stress, moods and chemicals associated with being overweight. Research has shown that low serotonin levels are associated with the craving for sweets and carbohydrates.

Stress has been shown to increase the level of cortisol which is linked to over-indulgence of simple carbohydrates such as chocolate, candy, sodas or ice cream. It has also been shown that when the body is stressed weight is conserved. The main ingredient in this category is 5-HTP otherwise known as "nature's serotonin." A common source of 5-HTP is Griffonia simplicifolia.

By replacing serotonin, cravings diminish and a general feeling of wellbeing is restored. This also helps reduce the stress in the body, thus having a positive impact on cortisol. Other ingredients commonly used include Hypericum perforatum (St. John's Wart) and Valerian root.

9. Influencing hormonal balance
It has been a common knowledge for a long time that hormonal imbalances can be directly related to weight gain. Low thyroid hormones is associated with weight gain, testosterone stimulates fat burning, and estrogen promotes fat storage. Information like this has led to research on other hormones as well.

We know there are certain hormones that affect satiety and hunger. However, there is a specific hormone that safely raises the resting metabolic rate. Although, this research is exciting and promising, finding natural and safe hormones that do not cause excess hormonal side effects is difficult.

The hormone leptin is the hormone of satiety and currently under study. Another hormone, 7-acetyl-3-oxo-dehydroepiandrosterone or 7-Keto is currently available and has been shown to safely raise the resting metabolic rate.

Although this is an exciting category, more research needs to be done.

10. Nutrition support

People who need to lose weight usually have a diet that lacks essential nutrients, vitamins, and minerals. It's important to support the body by overcoming deficiencies in things like antioxidants and essential fatty acids.

We always hear about cholesterol and the need to cut fats in the diet, but there's actually some essential fatty acids that you need to eat. Essential means the body doesn't make them, so you have to get them through your eating habits. Essential fatty acids improve cardiovascular health and the function of the body. (These are omega 3, 6 and 9) Another essential fatty acid are amino acids, the building blocks for the proteins that helps build your muscle, create lean muscle mass and decrease body fat.

Minerals such as potassium, calcium, magnesium, copper, zinc are very important too. Also, Fiber is needed as it helps suppress appetite, which decreases the overall caloric intake that promotes weight loss. Acai Berry is a well-documented ingredient which provides all of these nutritious elements. However, this shouldn't be misinterpreted as a primary weight loss ingredient.

"So Simon, what supplement should I get?"

Everybody's body is different regardless of how in-shape or out of shape they are. For instance, identical twins who weigh practically the same and partake in similar lifestyles could be deficient in different nutrients. However, to answer your question, its best to invest in a proven multivitamin that provides essential vitamins and minerals that most people are deficient in. When shopping for a multivitamin, make sure it provides these 20 nutrients:

1. **Cobalamin (Vitamin B12)** - building block red blood cell formation, neurological function, and DNA synthesis.
2. **Biotin (Vitamin B7)** – Helps metabolize fatty and amino acids

3. **Riboflavin (Vitamin B2)** – Essential in energy metabolism, and for the metabolism of fats, ketone bodies, carbohydrates, and proteins.
4. **Vitamin A** - helps bone development, immune system, vision, cell reproduction & strength.
5. **Vitamin E** – provides anti-oxidant benefits
6. **Niacin (Vitamin B3)** – *improves cholesterol*
7. **Vitamin D** - helps in building strong bones and teeth, as well as improving the strength and durability of both red and white blood cells.
8. **Thiamine (Vitamin B1)** – improves electrolytes within nerve and muscle cells
9. **Vitamin B6 (Pyridoxine)** – helps red blood cells and immune system function properly
10. **Vitamin C (Ascorbic Acid)** - Main component in the building of Collagen, which is essentially the microscopic stuff that holds our skin and ligaments tight and flexible, and helps heals our wounds.
11. **Calcium** - helps build strong, healthy bones and contract your muscles, expand and contract blood vessels.
12. **Iron** - Involved in the transportation of oxygen from blood cells to vital organs.
13. **Leucine** - a branch of amino acid that aids in repairing and building muscle tissues.
14. **Selenium** – Provides antioxidant benefits
15. **Copper** -   has antioxidant benefits and supports production of collagen
16. **Magnesium** – Enables energy production and controls blood sugar
17. **Zinc** - Your immune system needs it to effectively defend itself from viruses and bacteria.
18. **Chromium** – Essential for the production of insulin
19. **DHA** - Promotes healthy brain function
20. **Folate** - Helps new cells grow and helps old cells repair themselves.

Chapter 9: Is It Processed-Free? How Processed Foods Affect the Mind & Body

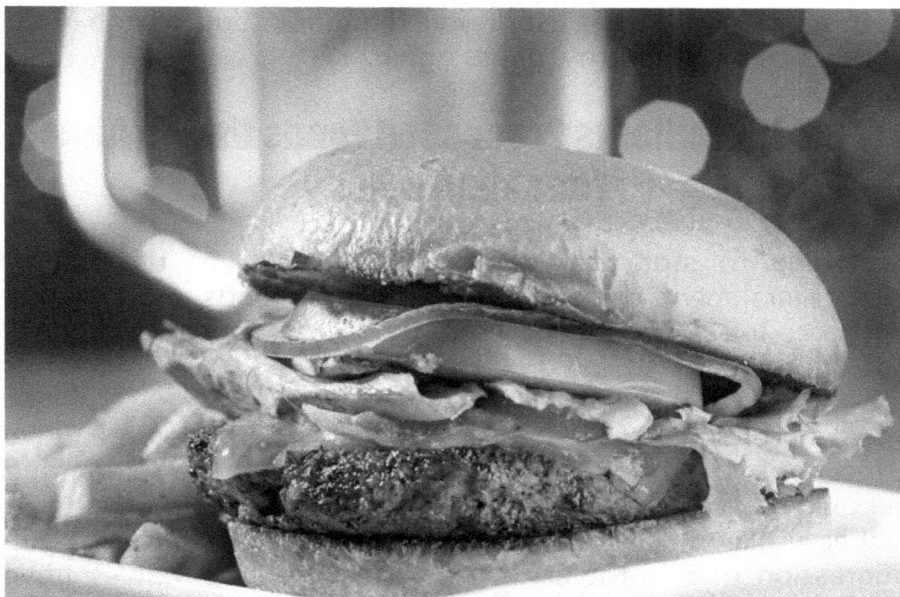

Forget gluten-free, make sure it is "processed-free!"

D id you know that some so-called gluten-free foods ACTUALLY contain trace amounts of gluten due to cross-contamination during processing? This is one of many revelations that many food companies would rather you not know. That's why my mantra is to ignore anything that's labeled gluten-free, sugar-free, fat-free, carb-free, or anything "free." As I mentioned several chapters ago, if a food is devoid of one substance, it contains an overabundance of another.

"Simon, what about non-GMO and organic labeled foods?"

Remember rule #13 of what fit, healthy individuals know...Everything labeled gluten-free and organic isn't healthy; the same goes for non-GMO foods. Another secret that food companies fail to disclose is that any food could be labeled "non-GMO" because it is unregulated. Therefore, anyone can claim that their product is non-GMO, because the FDA has not set any standards to regulate the use of this claim on a label. So if you thought a bag of non-GMO Dorito's chips is healthy, guess again.

The 3 Ingredients Processed Foods Use To Affect Your Mind & Body

According to statistics, approximiately 90% of the money Westerners spend on food is on processed foods. Most people are more likely to eat processed, laboratory foods vs. organic, natural food. That's sad.

Speaking of sad, these unnatural foods could have a negative effect on your mood. Researchers studied the diets and behaviors of nearly 1,000 men and women and found that a higher intake of trans fat was significantly tied to an increase in aggression and irritability. In addition, several studies have linked trans fat to heart disease, infertility, cancer, type 2 diabetes, liver problems, and of course... obesity.

Trans Fat

Food makers once used artificial trans fats to enhance the flavor, texture, and shelf life of processed foods; including packaged baked goods, snacks, and greasy fast food . Due to the FDA's recent abolishment of trans fat, most food companies have removed trans fat from there food. However, there are some food companies who sneakily label trans fat as "partially hydrogenated oils", yet claim to have zero grams of trans fat.

So please look at the nutrition label and ingredients to see if the product is truly devoid of trans fat.

High Fructose Corn Syrup (HFCS)

Processed foods are usually loaded with added sugar or its evil twin, HFCS. Remember when I briefly spoke about HFCS? In case you don't, here's a reminder of what my dear pal, Dr. Cola, had to say about processed food's favorite sweetener: *"The problem with high fructose corn syrup is that the brain does NOT recognize this as food, meaning that when we eat this, we don't feel full."* Of course, this is a big roadblock for weight loss.

"Simon, what exactly is HFCS?"

Cane sugar had been America's sweetener of choice for most of the 20th Century. Around late 1950s, High-Fructose Corn Syrup, derived from corn- sweeteners, was created by Japanese scientists. By the late 1960s & 1970s, due to its lower cost vs. cane sugar, HFCS was being frequently used as an ingredient in packaged food. While table sugar ratio of fructose to glucose is 1:1, HFCS ratio is 4:1, almost twice the fructose of common table sugar. Despite both containing four calories per gram, HFCS comes with 2 issues:

Issue #1: Your body cannot digest a ton of fructose

The reason for that is because metabolizing excess amounts of fructose is the major concern. The human body was meant to digest just a small amount of fructose while glucose derived from carbs we eat; therefore, your body can readily handle a good amount of glucose as it is able to release insulin to regulate glucose. (i.e., use it for fuel or energy).

On the other hand, fructose is processed by the liver. When excessive amounts of fructose enters the liver, it is unable to process quickly enough for the body to convert into energy. Instead, it creates fats from the fructose and sends them off into the bloodstream as triglycerides. To sum it up, too much triglyceride in your bloodstream over time increases your risk for heart disease, weight gain, and possibly type-2 diabetes.

Issue #2: Sugar is Sugar

Regardless, if a food or beverage consists of HFCS or cane sugar, it is still sugar. Too much sugar can cause a slew of health issues including cancer, obesity, diabetes, heart disease and metabolic syndrome. That's the problem processed food presents.

While more studies need to be conducted to further analyze the effects of HFCS, it's best you avoid any food or drink that has it listed as an ingredient.

Salt

Where there's sugar, there's salt. Anything that tastes sweet and salty is probably the epitome of an unnatural food or beverage. If you combine loads of sugar and salt with partially hydrogenated oil, you have the recipe for turning people to processed-food zombies...and I'm being serious. Some reports have shown that many people have become addicted to junk food. One study revealed that sugar and highly rewarding junk foods activate the same areas in the brain that drugs such as cocaine do.

Salt may be the worst of the three ingredients. Salt is the main reason that unnatural foods taste so yummy; that's how the food manufacturer successfully get people to buy their product.Too much sodium (i.e., salt) in your diet is very bad for your health. While the daily recommendation so sodium intake is about 1500 mg, the average American consumes 3400 mg of sodium per day or twice the amount that is recommended.

Here are some health risk factors that have been linked to a diet that consists of excess sodium intake:
- High Blood Pressure (or Hypertension)
- Stroke
- Heart Failure
- Kidney Stones
- Osteoporosis
- Kidney Disease
- Stomach Cancer
- Enlarged Heart Muscle

- Chronic Headaches

In addition, excess sodium affects your appearance by retaining water in which causes puffiness to certain body parts (legs, wrists, hands, feet), bloating of the stomach, and weight gain. Basically, excess water weight is usually attributed to excess sodium intake.

You want to know the crazy part about sodium? Your body needs it! While sodium has been heavily criticized in the mainstream media, it is a necessary mineral for your body to function properly. Here are the functions of sodium for your body:

- Facilitate muscle contraction and nerve cell transmission
- Helps maintain normal water balance
- Controls blood volume and blood pressure

The primary way to get dietary sodium is by ingesting salt through food & beverage consumption. Unfortunately, the western diet is now overloaded with sodium, especially processed foods.

Here are some tips on how to reduce sodium intake:

- Buy only fresh foods and vegetables instead of the canned versions
- Opt for fresh meat instead of packaged meat. Fresh cuts of beef, chicken or pork contain natural sodium while packaged meat contains a ton of sodium in order to preserve freshness. *(Note: If a meat item stays fresh in your fridge for weeks, it is likely because it has high sodium content)*
- Beware of products that do not taste salty but still have high sodium content, such as cottage cheese.
- <u>Learn how to eat food without adding salt</u>. It will take about 2 months for most people's taste buds to be adjusted to eating less sodium foods. Once your taste buds are adjusted, salty foods such as potato chips will taste saltier.
- Select spices or seasonings that do not list sodium (or salt) on their labels *(i.e. choose garlic powder over garlic salt)*
- <u>Limit going out to eat at restaurants</u>. Many restaurant foods are loaded with sodium. Conduct research about the restaurant beforehand to see which foods do not contain a ton of sodium.
- <u>Get 7-8 hours of quality sleep.</u> Research shows sleep deprivation leads most people to craving salty foods.

High sodium intake has gotten so rampant that the <u>FDA</u> has recently asked food makers and eating establishments to "voluntarily" reduce salt levels in their products to help reduce Americans' high salt intake. Do you think they will volunteer to do so? Not most of them. Most food companies won't reduce salt levels until the FDA regulates them do so as they did with trans-fat.

3 Unhealthy Things Processed Foods Provide

High Amounts of Refined Carbs (aka Bad Carbs)

There's a raging war in the health community about determining whether carbohydrates are good or bad for us. There are those that feel that carbs are essential for energy while other's feel it is detrimental to our livelihood. Well both sides are right....to a certain extent.

Carbs are designed to provide us with energy but it depends on the source. If the source is fruits, vegetables and sweet potatoes, then carbs are excellent. However, if the source derives from sugary cereal, Ho Ho cakes, and white bread, then carbs are horrible.

Processed foods provide refined (bad) carbs that are quickly broken down in the digestive tract, leading to rapid spikes in insulin levels and blood sugar. In addition, this leads people to feeling grumpy and tired immediately after eating these types of foods. But that's not all! Studies have linked refined carbs to the following health issues:

- Obesity
- Type-II Diabetes
- Heart Disease
- High Triglyceride Levels
- Overeating
- Colon Cancer
- Constipation & Other Digestive Problems

If these risk factors don't make you think twice before ordering pizza, then what will?

Low Amount of Nutrients

In the last chapter, I mentioned how supplements wasn't a magic pill. The main reason it isn't is because your body craves real, whole foods for its nutrients; supplements ONLY assist the body in getting those nutrients. With that said you cannot eat mostly processed, un-nutritious foods and expect a multivitamin to take care of the rest. It doesn't work that way.

To make up for the lack of nutrients, some food companies have the audacity to add artificial vitamins and minerals to food during processing. Of course, these artificial nutrients are not a good replacement for the real ones found in whole food. Another factor is; there are thousands of nutrients within whole foods that health researchers are yet to uncover. Overall, its best you opt for chicken instead of chicken nuggets to get more nutrients.

Low Amount of Fiber

The reason refined carbs causes constipation and other digestive problems is due to low fiber content. Fiber (especially soluble fiber) is very beneficial to your body. It acts as a prebiotic, which cleanses the gut by providing the intestine with friendly bacteria. In addition, research has shown that fiber could slow absorption of carbs, helping you feel satisfied off less calories.

Processed foods messes all of that up. During processing, foods that normally provides fiber is removed or lost (e.g. bread); this leaves the foods with little to no fiber left. So, if you are having a hard time with bowel movements, you can thank processed foods for that.

Chapter 10: 7-Day Colon Cleanse Detox.... With Real Food

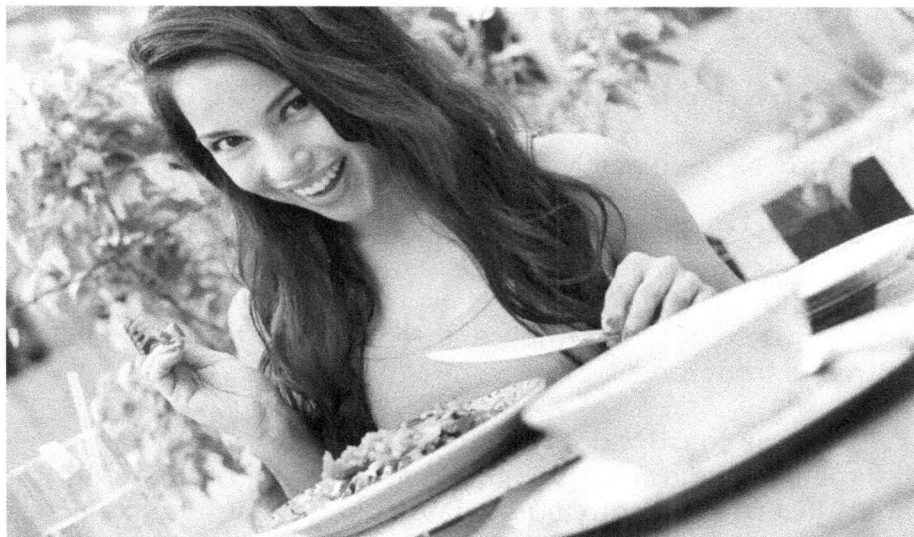

Now it's time for some action! It is time to get your body ready for this new healthy lifestyle. In other words, it's time to clean out the gunk by doing this 7-day colon cleanse detox! Unlike other cleanses, this one utilize real foods so, no, you won't be consuming just soup and tea.

Not sure if you need a cleanse? Well your system definitely needs some "spring cleaning" if you exhibit one or more of the following symptoms:

- Overweight/Obese
- Bloating
- Constipation
- Low Energy Levels
- Poor Appetite
- Backaches

- Diarrhea
- Stinky Breath
- Headaches
- Mood Swings
- Weak Immune System (i.e., Get sick easily)

If you are nodding your head right now, then it is time for a colon cleanse detox. For centuries, people have gotten their colon cleansed for a variety of reasons.

Here are the 5 benefits of getting yours cleansed:

1. Improves the digestive system function

If you've been feeling clogged up like an ancient toilet, then a colon cleanses is what you need. By cleansing your colon, you remove harmful waste from your digestive system. Detoxification makes it easier for body to absorb nutrients from food.

2. Relieves constipation
Let me be candid for a sec: It is not fun being on the toilet for hours just to eventually barely poop out almost nothing. If that is your current situation, it is time get your colon cleansed ASAP.

3. Boost energy levels
When you are clogged up and constipated, that zaps your energy. The toxins left by undigested waste are the reason for that. By getting your colon cleansed, it releases the toxins in your body; thus, boosting your energy levels.

4. Improves mental focus & thinking
Been having brain fart issues, lately? Well you can thank your clogged up colon for that! Toxic matter in your body mentally affects your ability to focus and think. Detoxing clears up the brain to properly function.

5. Aid weight loss efforts
Probably the most popular benefit of detoxification is it helps you lose weight. When you are unclogged (i.e., more bowel

movements), have more energy to exercise, and able to absorb nutrients better, it makes sense how a detox can help you lose some weight. Don't you think?

7 Days Colon Cleanse Detox Plan

Our body produces many toxic products and substances daily. Our body needs to be detoxified of these products in order to work efficiently. There are many ways to detoxify these harmful substances. Natural and innate ways are the key to detoxification process and our body gets rid of toxic substances by some natural ways like sweating, respiration, urination and defecation.

There are various ways to speed up these processes.... this 7-day cleanse is one of them.

This 7-day cleanse ensures that your system is not only cleansed, but ready to transition to a healthier lifestyle. Below you find the shopping list of foods you need along with the 7-day cleanse meal plan.

Shopping list:
- Lemon
- Eggs
- Pepper
- Honey
- Vegetables for salad: broccoli, beetroot, cabbage, radish, carrot, cauliflower, lettuce, onions, tomatoes and turnips
- Apple Cider vinegar
- Fruits: apples, plums, asparagus, banana, strawberry, raspberry, squash, pineapples, kiwifruit, grapes, grapefruit, melons
- Avocado
- Potato and sweet potatoes
- Brown rice
- Lemon grass tea
- Honey
- Ginger
- Garlic

- Fresh yogurt
- Lime
- Brown rice
- Walnut
- Protein Powder
- Organic turkey
- Wild caught sea bass
- Organic chicken
- Wild-caught mahi mahi
- Wild-caught tuna
- Wild-caught swordfish
- Eggs
- Wild-caught tilapia
- Organic Baking mix
- Wild caught swordfish

Detox Green Tea Recipe:

Ingredients:
- 1 cup Hot water
- 1 tsp. Powdered ginger
- 1 tsp. apple cider vinegar
- 1 tsp. Organic Cayenne
- Squeezed organic lemon

7-Day Cleanse Meal Plan
Note: Grill or baked the chicken, fish and turkey

Day 1:
Upon waking: Detox green tea
Breakfast:4 boiled eggs, Mixed grain porridge drizzled with honey and walnuts

Snack: Organic turkey (3.5 OZ.), Fresh juice of your choice,

Lunch: Organic chicken (4 OZ), vegetable salad with pepper and honey, Rice cakes topped with Olive
Snack: Protein shake, figs or dates if you are hungry
Supper: Wild caught sea bass (3.5 OZ.), Vegetable platter

Bed time: Hot water, Homemade yogurt, Fruit Salad

Day 2:
Upon waking: Detox green tea
Breakfast: Protein shake and fruit platter
Snack: 2 boiled eggs, Handful of sunflower seeds, Fresh juice
Lunch: Wild-caught tuna (3.5 OZ.), fruit platter
Snack: Protein powder, fresh fruits such as avocado, figs, etc.
Supper: Wild caught mahi mahi (3.5 oz), Avocado salad with bell peppers and grape fruit
Bed time: Hot water with honey

Day 3:
Upon waking: Detox green tea
Breakfast: Protein shake
Snack: Organic chicken (3.5 OZ.), fresh juice of your choice
Lunch: Wild caught tilapia (3.5 OZ.), vegetable platter
Snack: 2 Boiled eggs, Lemon juice
Supper: Organic turkey (3.5 OZ), beet root salad with cucumber and broccoli and mashed potatoes
Bed time: hot water

Day 4:
On waking: Detox green tea
Breakfast: Nutty muesli topped with homemade yogurt, Fruit Platte
Snack: 2 boiled eggs, one banana and handful of nuts
Lunch: Wild-caught sea bass, 1 or 2 fresh fruits of your choice
Snack: Wild caught swordfish (4.5OZ), Fresh fruit juice
Supper: Wild caught tuna (4.0 oz.), cucumber 1 cup, beet root ½ cup, melon 1 cup
Bed time: Hot water

Day 5:
On waking: Detox green tea
Breakfast: Protein powder (4 oz.), Organic blue berries
Snack: Organic turkey (4oz), a handful of your favorite nuts
Lunch: Organic chicken salad, Mineral water
Tea time: fresh lime, fresh fruit if feel hungry
Supper: Vegetable soup, boiled eggs
Bed time: Hot water

Day 6:
Upon waking: Detox green tea
Breakfast: Homemade yogurt, Wild-caught Swordfish (4 oz.), fresh juice of your choice
Snack: 2 boiled eggs, dates and figs
Lunch: Brown rice with yogurt, 1 generous portion of Vegetable Salad
Supper: Carrot and cucumber soup, Wild Caught Mahi Mahi
Bed time: Hot water

Day 7:
Upon Waking: Detox Green tea
Breakfast: Protein powder, Fruit salad platter
Snack: Wild caught tilapia (4.5 oz.), fresh fruits such as apple and pear
Lunch: Potato and celery salad with walnuts, Salad plate
Tea time: Green tea, handful of nuts
Supper: Organic chicken (4 oz.), Vegetable salad plate
Bed time: Hot water

Section 4: Fat Burning Exercise

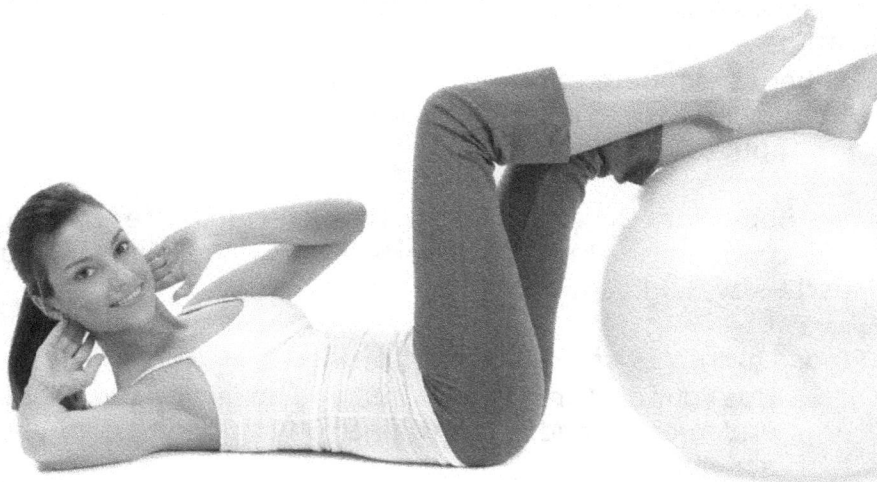

Chapter 11: Exercise Questionnaire

Finally, it is time to burn some fat and lose weight.... well not quite. Before we embark on the exercise program, please take this questionnaire that will analyze your exercise readiness. It should take no longer than 10 minutes to complete, so, please take your time and answer each question honestly.

Note: If you decide to hire a personal trainer, these questions will help them determine where you are at health-wise.

What do you wish to get out of exercise? Please circle all options that applies.

Lose Body Fat, Develop Muscle Tone, Rehabilitate an Injury, Start an Exercise Program, Sports Specific Training, Increase Muscle Size, Fun, Motivation

Please mark YES or No to the following:

1. Has your doctor ever said that you have a heart condition and recommended only medically supervised physical activity? _____
2. Do you frequently have pains in your chest when you perform physical activity? _____
3. Have you had chest pain when you were not doing physical activity? _____
4. Do you lose your balance due to dizziness or do you ever lose consciousness? _____
5. Do you have a bone, joint or any other health problem that causes you pain or limitations that must be addressed when developing an exercise program (i.e. diabetes, osteoporosis, high blood pressure, high cholesterol, arthritis, anorexia, bulimia, anemia,

epilepsy, respiratory ailments, back problems, etc.)?
_____

6. Are you pregnant now or have given birth within the last 6 months? _____
7. Have you had a recent surgery? _____
8. Do you take any medications, either prescription or non-prescription, on a regular basis? Yes/No
9. If yes, what is the medication for?
_____
_____

10. How does this medication affect your ability to exercise or achieve your fitness goals?
_____
_____

Note: If you answered **YES** to any of the aforementioned questions, please talk with your doctor by phone or in person BEFORE you start becoming much more physically active or BEFORE you have a fitness assessment or program.

Lifestyle Related Questions:
1) Do you smoke? YES/ NO If yes, how many times per day?
_____
2) Do you drink alcohol? YES/ NO If yes, how many glasses per week?_____
3) How many hours do you regularly sleep at night?
_____
4) Describe your job: Sedentary Active   Physically Demanding
5) Does your job require travel? YES/ NO
6) On a scale of 1-10, how would you rate your stress level (1=very low 10=very high)? _____
7) List your 3 biggest sources of stress:
a. _____   b. _____
c._____
8) Is anyone in your immediate family overweight? Mother Father Sibling(s) Grandparent(s)
9) Were you overweight as a child? YES NO If yes, at what age(s)?
_____

Fitness History:
1) When were you in the best shape of your life?
_____
2) Have you been exercising consistently for the past 3 months?
YES NO
3) When did you first start thinking about getting in shape?
_____
4) What if anything stopped you in the past?
_____
5) On a scale of 1-10, how would you rate your present fitness level (1=Worst 10=Best)? _____

Exercise Related Questions: (Skip to next section if you are physically inactive)
1) How often do you take part in physical exercise? (Check one)
5-7x/week 3-4x/week 1-2x/week
2) If your participation is lower than you would like it to be, what are the reasons?
Lack of Interest Illness/Injury Lack of Time Other (Please specify)
_____
3) How long have you been consistently physically active for?
_____
4) What physical activities are you currently involved in? (Check all that applies)

Walking Jogging Running Weightlifting Yoga Sports Other (Please specify) _____

Developing your Fitness Program:
1. Please circle how you prefer to exercise:
a) INSIDE, OUTSIDE, or COMBINATION
b) LARGE GROUPS, SMALL GROUPS, ALONE, or COMBINATION
c) MORNING, AFTERNOON, or EVENING
d) HOME, GYM, or OUTSIDE
2. Realistically, how often a week would you like to exercise?
_____x/week
3. Realistically, how much time would you like to spend during each exercise session? _____
4. What are the best days during the week for you to commit to an exercise program?
Monday Tuesday Wednesday Thursday Friday Saturday Sunday

Goal Setting:
1. Please list in order of priority, the fitness goals you would like to achieve in the next 3 to 12 months?
a)
_____
b)
_____
c)
_____

2. How will you feel once you've achieved these goals? Be specific.
_____
_____
_____
_____

3. Where do you rate health your life? Low priority Medium Priority High priority
4. HONESTLY, how committed are you to achieving your fitness goals? Very Semi   Not very
5. Briefly explain what you feel are the obstacles or your potential actions, behaviors or activities that could impede your progress towards accomplishing your goals (i.e. not training consistently, upcoming vacation, busy season at work, not following the program, allowing other responsibilities to become a priority over exercise etc.).
_____
_____
_____
_____
_____

6. Outline 3 methods that you plan to use to overcome these obstacles:
a. _____
b. _____
c._____

Chapter 12: Simon's 1-Month Training Guide

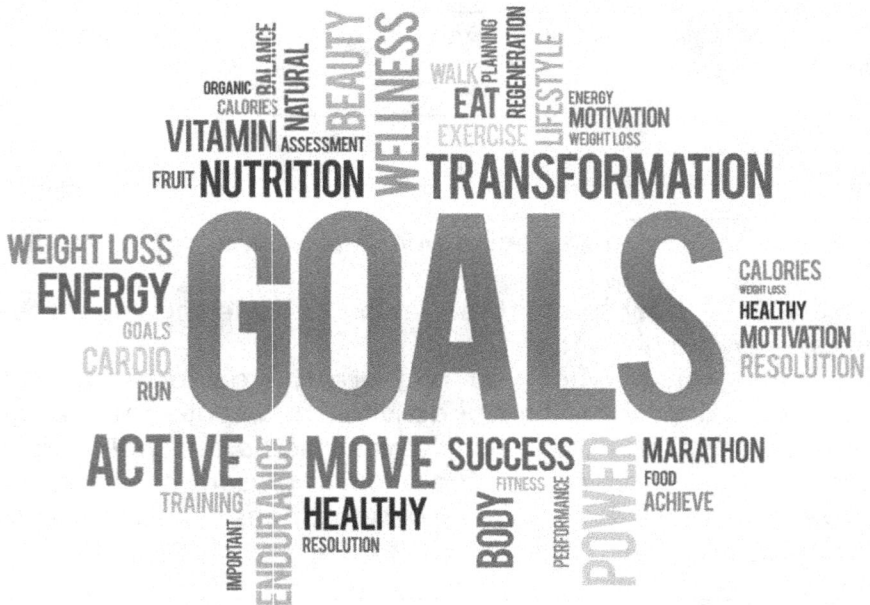

Now, it is time to exercise! Since I have no clue what type of exercise you like to do, I decided to whip up a 1-month fat-burning exercise routine for you to do 4 days per week; it combines weightlifting and bodyweight exercises to work your entire physique.

To perform this 1-month sample routine, please get a gym membership if you don't already have one. On your non-training days, I recommend doing low-intense activities such as taking a yoga class, walking, or partaking in an activity with family/friends (e.g., sports, hiking, etc.)

So are you ready ignite fat and lose some weight? Well start training today!

Note: If 4 days of training is too intense for you, then only train 3 days per week; ideally on Monday, Wednesday, and Friday.

Training Frequency
You will train 4 days per week. In this sample training guideline, the training days at the gym will be on Monday, Tuesday, Thursday, and Friday. Wednesday, Saturday and Sunday are active rest days. Chose whatever 4 days you have at least 45 minutes to 1 hour to train.

Exercise Guidelines
Some exercises that are performed with weights will based off a percentage of your 1-rep max (1RM). For example, you are prescribed to do bench press for 3 x 10 (75% 1RM) with a 90 seconds rest. That means that you do 10 reps for 3 sets with a weight that is 75% of your 1 rep max and rest 90 seconds between sets. Each exercise will help engage in movements that helps you burn a great amount of calories.

Week 1 Training

Week 1 Training Routine (Monday)
Warm-up Routine (do each exercise in order for 1 minute)
- Jog in place
- Jumping Jacks
- Lunge Walks
- Arm Circles

Exercise:	Dumbbell Chest Press	Barbell Squats	Pushups*	Burpees	Jump Rope
Sets and Reps:	3 x 10 reps	3 x 10 reps	3 x 15 to 20 reps	3 x 12 to 15 reps	5 x 30 secs
Rest time:	90 seconds	90 secs	60 secs	60 secs	30 secs
% of 1RM:	70%	70%	Bodyweight	Bodyweight	Bodyweight

* Do pushups on your knees if unable to do regular pushups

Week 1 Training Routine (Tuesday)
Warm-up Routine (do each exercise in order for 1 minute)
- Jog in place
- Jumping Jacks
- Lunge Walks
- Arm Circles

Exercise:	Pull-ups*	Dumbbell Lunges	One-arm dumbbell row	Kettlebell Swings	Mountain Climbers
Sets and Reps:	3 x 10 reps	3 x 10 reps	3 x 12 to 15 reps	3 x 15 to 20 reps	5 x 30 secs
Rest time:	90 seconds	90 secs	60 secs	60 secs	30 secs
% of 1RM:	Bodyweight	70%	60%	50%	Bodyweight

*Use assisted pull-up machine if unable to do regular pull-ups

Week 1 Training Routine (Wednesday)
Walk 2 miles today outside or on a treadmill (put on incline 3 if on using treadmill)
Week 1 Training Routine (Thursday)
Warm-up Routine (do each exercise in order for 1 minute)
- Jog in place
- Jumping Jacks
- Lunge Walks
- Arm Circles

Exercise:	Dumbbell Chest Press	Barbell Squats	Pushups*	Burpees	Jump Rope
Sets and Reps:	3 x 12 reps	3 x 12 reps	3 x 15 to 20 reps	3 x 12 to 15 reps	6 x 30 secs
Rest time:	90 seconds	90 secs	60 secs	60 secs	30 secs
% of 1RM:	70%	70%	Bodyweight	Bodyweight	Bodyweight

* Do pushups on your knees if unable to do regular pushups

Week 1 Training Routine (Friday)

Warm-up Routine (do each exercise in order for 1 minute)

- Jog in place
- Jumping Jacks
- Lunge Walks
- Arm Circles

Exercise:	Pull-ups*	Dumbbell Lunges	One-arm dumbbell row	Kettlebell Swings	Mountain Climbers
Sets and Reps:	3 x 11 reps	3 x 12 reps	3 x 12 to 15 reps	3 x 15 to 20 reps	5 x 30 secs
Rest time:	90 seconds	90 secs	60 secs	60 secs	30 secs
% of 1RM:	Bodyweight	70%	60%	50%	Bodyweight

*Use assisted pull-up machine if unable to do regular pull-ups

Week 1 Training Routine (Saturday)

Do 20-30 minutes of yoga to help soothe your achy muscles.

Week 1 Training Routine (Sunday)

Just completely relax. Kick back and watch TV, play solitaire, read gossip sites or whatever relaxing hobby will put you at ease.

Week 2 Training

Week 2 Training Routine (Monday)
Warm-up Routine (do each exercise in order for 1 minute)
- Jog in place
- Jumping Jacks
- Lunge Walks
- Arm Circles

Exercise:	Dumbbell Chest Press	Barbell Squats	Cable Chest Press	Lateral Hops*	Sprint Intervals on Treadmill**
Sets and Reps:	3 x 10 reps	3 x 10 reps	3 x 15 to 20 reps	3 x 15 reps	6 x 30 secs
Rest time:	90 seconds	90 secs	60 secs	60 secs	30 secs
% of 1RM:	75%	75%	65%	Bodyweight	Bodyweight

** Completing a hop on both sides counts as 1 rep
*Put treadmill incline on 3 and walk during the rest time

Week 2 Training Routine (Tuesday)
Warm-up Routine (do each exercise in order for 1 minute)
- Jog in place
- Jumping Jacks
- Lunge Walks
- Arm Circles

Exercise:	Pull-ups	Dumbbell Lunges	One-arm dumbbell row	Bear Crawls*	Run up a hill**
Sets and Reps:	3 x 12 reps	3 x 13 reps	3 x 12 to 15 reps	3 x 20 yards	5 x 30 secs
Rest time:	90 seconds	90 secs	60 secs	60 seconds	60 secs
% of 1RM:	Bodyweight	70%	65%	Bodyweight	Bodyweight

*Find an open field that has 20 yards of open space
**Find a slope hill to run up

Week 2 Training Routine (Wednesday)
Walk 2 miles. (If too easy, hold a pair of 3lb dumbbells doing the movement)

Week 2 Training Routine (Thursday)
Warm-up Routine (do each exercise in order for 1 minute)
- Jog in place
- Jumping Jacks
- Lunge Walks
- Arm Circles

Exercise:	Dumbbell Chest Press	Barbell Squats	Cable Chest Press	Lateral Hops*	Sprint Intervals on Treadmill**
Sets and Reps:	3 x 12 reps	3 x 12 reps	3 x 15 to 20 reps	3 x 15 reps	6 x 30 secs
Rest time:	90 seconds	90 secs	60 secs	60 secs	30 secs
% of 1RM:	75%	75%	65%	Bodyweight	Bodyweight

** Completing a hop on both sides counts as 1 rep
*Put treadmill incline on 3 and walk during the rest time

Week 2 Training Routine (Friday)
Warm-up Routine (do each exercise in order for 1 minute)
- Jog in place
- Jumping Jacks
- Lunge Walks

Exercise:	Pull-ups	Dumbbell Lunges	One-arm dumbbell row	Bear Crawls*	Run up a hill**
Sets and Reps:	3 x 12 reps	3 x 13 reps	3 x 12 to 15 reps	3 x 20 yards	5 x 30 secs
Rest time:	90 seconds	90 secs	60 secs	60 seconds	60 secs
% of 1RM:	Bodyweight	70%	65%	Bodyweight	Bodyweight

Week 2 Training Routine (Saturday)
Yoga time!

Week 2 Training Routine (Sunday)
- Arm Circles

*Find an open field that has 20 yards of open space
**Find a slope hill to run up
Relax time! You deserve it!

Week 3 Training

Week 3 Training Routine (Monday)
Warm-up Routine (do each exercise in order for 1 minute)
- Jog in place
- Jumping Jacks
- Lunge Walks
- Arm Circles

Exercise:	Dumbbell Chest Press	Barbell Squats	Decline Pushups	Step-ups*	Mountain Climbers
Sets and Reps:	4 x 8 reps	3 x 15-20 reps	3 x 10 reps	3 x 20 reps	5 x 40 secs
Rest time:	120 seconds	90 secs	60 secs	60 secs	40 secs
% of 1RM:	80%	70%	Bodyweight	Bodyweight	Bodyweight

* Do prescribed reps for each leg

Week 3 Training Routine (Tuesday)
Warm-up Routine (do each exercise in order for 1 minute)
- Jog in place
- Jumping Jacks
- Lunge Walks
- Arm Circles

Exercise:	Pull-ups*	Dumbbell Lunges	One-arm dumbbell row	Jump Rope**	Run up a hill***
Sets and Reps:	4 x 8 reps	3 x 8 reps	3 x 10-12 reps	5 x 30 seconds	5 x 30 secs
Rest time:	120 seconds	90 secs	60 secs	30 seconds	60 secs
% of 1RM:	Bodyweight	80%	70%	Bodyweight	Bodyweight

*Pause at the top position for 2-4 seconds
**Jump rope fast as possible for prescribed seconds
***Find an open hill or do this on a treadmill (set incline to 5)

Week 3 Training Routine (Wednesday)
Pick a leisure activity that involves walking for 1 hour (e.g. walk your dog, go the mall, etc.)
Week 3 Training Routine (Thursday)
Warm-up Routine (do each exercise in order for 1 minute)

- Jog in place
- Jumping Jacks
- Lunge Walks
- Arm Circles

Exercise:	Dumbbell Chest Press	Barbell Squats	Decline Pushups	Step-ups*	Mountain Climbers
Sets and Reps:	4 x 10 reps	3 x 12-15 reps	3 x 12 reps	3 x 20 reps	5 x 40 secs
Rest time:	120 seconds	90 secs	60 secs	60 secs	40 secs
% of 1RM:	80%	75%	Bodyweight	Bodyweight	Bodyweight

* Do prescribed reps for each leg

Week 3 Training Routine (Friday)
Warm-up Routine (do each exercise in order for 1 minute)
- Jog in place
- Jumping Jacks
- Lunge Walks
- Arm Circles

Exercise:	Pull-ups*	Dumbbell Lunges	One-arm dumbbell row	Jump Rope**	Run up a hill***
Sets and Reps:	4 x 10 reps	3 x 10 reps	3 x 10-12 reps	5 x 30 seconds	5 x 30 secs
Rest time:	120 seconds	90 secs	60 secs	30 seconds	60 secs
% of 1RM:	Bodyweight	80%	70%	Bodyweight	Bodyweight

*Pause at the top position for 2-4 seconds
**Jump rope fast as possible for prescribed seconds
***Find an open hill or do this on a treadmill (set incline to 5)

Week 3 Training Routine (Saturday)
Get with friends and play a sport (e.g. basketball, flag football, etc.)
Week 3 Training Routine (Sunday)
Relax and unwind. Catch up on your favorite TV shows!

Week 4 Training

Week 4 Training Routine (Monday)
Warm-up Routine (do each exercise in order for 1 minute)
- Jog in place
- Jumping Jacks
- Lunge Walks
- Arm Circles

Exercise:	Dumbbel l Chest Press	Barbel l Squat s	Cabl e Ches t Press	Bear Crawls*	Sprints**
Sets and Reps:	4 x 12 reps	3 x 12-15 reps	3 x 20-30 reps	3 x 20 yards	5 x 20 yards
Rest time:	120 seconds	60 secs	60 secs	60 secs	60 secs
% of 1RM:	80%	70%	60%	Bodyweigh t	Bodyweigh t

*find open field to perform bear crawls
**Find open field or track to perform sprints

Week 4 Training Routine (Tuesday)
Warm-up Routine (do each exercise in order for 1 minute)
- Jog in place
- Jumping Jacks
- Lunge Walks
- Arm Circles

Exercise:	Pull-ups*	Jump Squats	Cable Row	Burpees	Lateral Hops
Sets and Reps:	4 x 12 reps	3 x 15-20 reps	3 x 12-15 reps	5 x 12-15 seconds	5 x 30 secs
Rest time:	120 seconds	60 secs	60 secs	60 seconds	60 secs
% of 1RM:	Bodyweight	Bodyweight	60%	Bodyweight	Bodyweight

*Pause at the top position for 2-4 seconds

Week 4 Training Routine (Wednesday)
Do some yoga.

Week 4 Training Routine (Thursday)
Warm-up Routine (do each exercise in order for 1 minute)
- Jog in place
- Jumping Jacks
- Lunge Walks
- Arm Circles

Exercise:	Dumbbell Chest Press	Barbell Squats	Cable Chest Press	Bear Crawls*	Sprints**
Sets and Reps:	4 x 15-20 reps	3 x 10-12 reps	3 x 20-30 reps	3 x 20 yards	5 x 20 yards
Rest time:	120 seconds	60 secs	60 secs	60 secs	60 secs
% of 1RM:	70%	75%	60%	Bodyweight	Bodyweight

*find open field to perform bear crawls
**Find open field or track to perform sprints

Week 4 Training Routine (Friday)
Warm-up Routine (do each exercise in order for 1 minute)
- Jog in place

- Jumping Jacks
- Lunge Walks
- Arm Circles

Exercise:	Pull-ups*	Jump Squats	Cable Row	Burpees	Lateral Hops
Sets and Reps:	4 x 12 reps	3 x 15-20 reps	3 x 12-15 reps	5 x 12-15 seconds	5 x 30 secs
Rest time:	90 seconds	60 secs	60 secs	60 seconds	60 secs
% of 1RM:	bodyweight	bodyweight	60%	bodyweight	Bodyweight

*Pause at the top position for 2-4 seconds

Week 4 Training Routine (Saturday)
Find an activity to do with your family members and/or friends (e.g. throwing a Frisbee, playing softball, etc.)
Week 4 Training Routine (Sunday)
Relax! As a matter of fact, go get a massage. You deserve it!

Conclusion

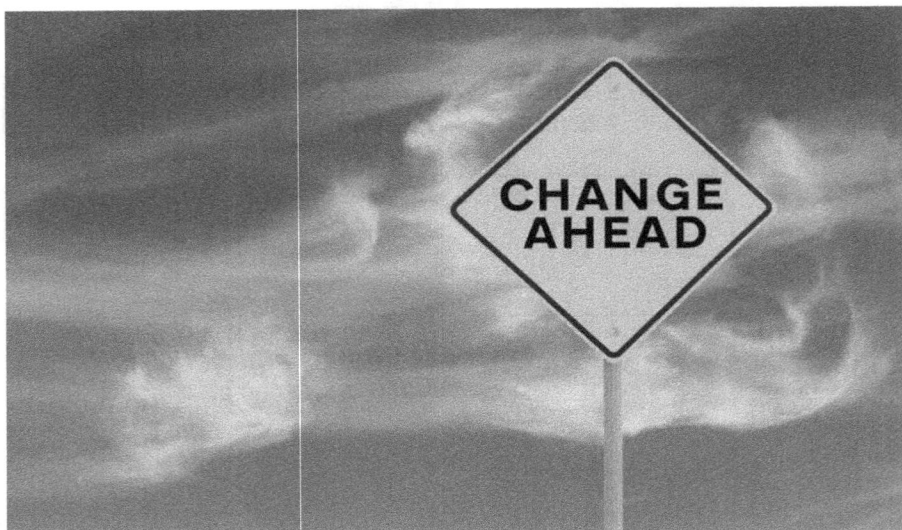

Phew!

Right now, you're probably feeling a bit overwhelmed. This book is not exactly what I would consider light reading. You've just completed a full-on immersion course on how to lose body fat, and you should be feeling proud of yourself. Feeling overwhelmed is actually a good thing because even though you feel like all that information is a big jumbles MESS upstairs, your brain is subconsciously making connections.

Right now, without you doing anything it's figuring out which part of your routine you should start on next? It's figuring out whether you need a supplement or not. It's wondering where to go for support/mentoring/accountability. All this is happening even though you may feel overwhelmed.

So what in the world should you do first? Here's what I recommend:
1. What is your weight loss goal? Decide on one right now.
2. Figure out when you want to get there (make it achievable or you won't even get to the start line) – and I mean write the date where you can see it every day!

3. Start your journey one step at a time – remember you need to combine the steps for both mind and body to make it happen (*e.g. Don't start the 7-day detox or workout program until you're 100% ready*)

This is a weight loss reference book. Don't read it once and go on with your business as usual, keep it handy and refer to it often when you need motivation – Think about the life and body you want to have. Dare to dream about how wonderful you will look and feel as you make changes.

Ignite your Weight Loss
I showed this book to a lot of people before it went to print , and many suggested I set up a coaching program or personal fitness business. Believe me, I thought long and hard about it. Remember my story? I spent such a long time researching the industry and saw first hand how many unqualified people are posing to be experts and succeeding in making millions off helpless victims like you and me?

Your body is an amazing, wonderful machine. No matter what shape you are in right now you can, with a few adjustments, create the best, most powerful and healthy version of you possible. Wouldn't that be great? Of course it would.

Humans are creatures of habit. No matter how disappointed you have been with previous results – you now have the ability to see dramatic changes in your physique when you understand how the tools I have laid out in this book can work for you.

It all comes down to the correct nutrition and training for YOUR body, for YOUR lifestyle – not mine or anyone else's – Just Yours. So I have created a resource for you to USE and SUPPORT and INSPIRE you to ignite your transformation and find out what your body is capable of.

- Simple, No BS proven information from experts
- Simple Nutritious recipes (for food choices you will enjoy and not dread)
- Latest fitness tips and tricks

- A support system to keep you on track so that you succeed

You can find it here:
http://feelfit.online/
Go Ignite Your Weightloss!
Thank you so much for reading this book and I wish you all the success you can dream of...

- Simon Brett

References

1. http://jamanetwork.com/journals/jama/article-abstract/202339
2. http://onlinelibrary.wiley.com/doi/10.1111/j.1467-789X.2008.00518.x/abstract
3. http://nutritionandmetabolism.biomedcentral.com/articles/10.1186/1743-7075-2-5
4. http://ajcn.nutrition.org/content/86/4/899.short
5. https://www.ncbi.nlm.nih.gov/pubmed/22011680
6. http://journals.lww.com/co-clinicalnutrition/Abstract/2010/07000/Neurobiology_of_food_addiction.3.aspx
7. http://ajcn.nutrition.org/content/76/1/266S.short
8. https://www.ncbi.nlm.nih.gov/pubmed/18287346
9. https://www.ncbi.nlm.nih.gov/pubmed/16387724'
10. http://ajcn.nutrition.org/content/66/4/1006S.short

www.ingramcontent.com/pod-product-compliance
Lightning Source LLC
Chambersburg PA
CBHW050540280326
41933CB00011B/1657